HERBS TO HELP YOU HEAL

Printed and Bound in the United States of America
Published and Distributed by:
Milligan Books, Inc.
1425 W. Manchester Avenue, Suite "C"
Los Angeles, California 90047
(323) 750-3592
Web site: www.milliganbooks.com

Cover Design: Kevin Allen

Formatting: Milligan Books

Second Printing , November 2009

10 9 8 7 6 5 4 3 2 1

ISBN 978-0-615-19812-5

www.herbstohelpyouheal.com

HERBS TO HELP YOU HEAL

Sylvia Gill

MILLIGAN BOOKS,INC.

BOOKS

CALIFORNIA

INTRODUCTION

TWELVE YEARS AGO I WAS diagnosed with breast cancer; at that time I begin researching herbs to help me heal; there were many herb books on the market as well as herbalist that I found helpful and enlightening. In my search I needed a quick reference that listed both the illness and the herbs together. I found no such book; I had to go in and out of the index of many books to find the herbs that I needed. That task brought about the beginning of this book. Once I discovered the herbs to use, I found there were many herbs that I could not take because of my high blood pressure. In this book I have tried to inform the reader of which herbs they are. There are herbs that people with diabetes should not use. This book will let you know which herbs not to take. Pregnant women should not take certain herbs during pregnancy and those herbs are also listed in this book. I needed to know how to prepare the herbs; there is a variety of ways in which to use and prepare these herbs. Capsules will take a longer time to get into the system before they begin to offer the results. For quicker results herbs is best taken as a tea. If preparing tea is not convenient, using juice that is without sugar can be used. It offers the same quick results as the tea. This book offers a suggested amount of how much of the herb to use at one time. Herbs may be taken for as long as you feel the need. However, it is best to take them in intervals, as an on and off procedure. After consulting several herbalists I realized this information might differ according to the individual. This book is designed to be a quick reference alphabetically connecting the ailment or the disease to the herb.

Each herbalist that I received information from had different opinions for the amount of herb to use, or for how long to use the herb; so this book offers a suggested amount of how much of the herb to take at once and for how long to take it which will differ one from another and may be altered in any way that is desired by the in-taker. This book also suggests that sugar or sodas, not be used to sweeten the tea or the juice of the herbs because it will inhibit the performance of the herb. For serious ailments it is best to use a juicer for preparing your juice.

In addition to the herbs listed in this book a healthy nutritional intake is most important. The nutritional intake may differ according to each individual. Sugar and alcohol of any kind will inhibit the benefit of taking these herbs during the time you are using them.

It is important to stress the herbs listed in this book is not intended to replace medications of any kind. Nor is it suggested to offer cures of any kind. It is important that professional help be consulted for an early diagnosis of an illness or disease. However, the knowledge of knowing that a disease is within your family; herbs may be beneficial for prevention, or a prolonged contact from the disease.

The herbs listed in this book with the asterisk (*) in front of the BOLD print is most highly beneficial for that particular ailment or disease listed in this book.

DISCLAIMER

It is important to stress that the herbs listed in this book is not intended to replace medications of any kind. Nor is it suggested to offer cures of any kind. It is important that professional help be consulted for an early diagnosis of an illness or disease. However, the knowledge of knowing that a disease exist within your family; herbs may be beneficial for prevention, or a prolonged contact from the disease providing they are taken at an early stage.

In addition to the herbs listed in this book a healthy nutritional intake is most important while dealing with health issues. The nutritional intake may differ according to each individual. Sugar and alcohol of any kind will inhibit the benefit of taking these herbs during the time you are using them.

ACKNOWLEDMENTS

This book is dedicated to my mother Ada Hill, my daughter Diane Landrum, my son Anthony Aburto, Sr., my nine beautiful grandchildren Adrin Davis, Katrina Parham, Yesenia Aburto, Anthony Aburto, Jr. Imara Aburto Long, Liana Aburto, Christina Aburto, Monica Aburto, Noelle Santa Maria-Aburto, and my fifteen great grandchildren. Thanks to my brother Joseph Hill; my sisters Barbara Kelley; and Carol Lampkins.

Thanks to my nieces; Shanti Hill; Kyla Hill; Renee Davis; Rhonda Ann Lockhart; and my late niece Brigette Hill. Thanks to my nephews Byron Hill; and Yusaf Hill. Many of who call me whenever there is a need for herbs.

This is a Special love to my late son Edward (Eddie) Aburto who waited six months before telling me that he had a lump in his neck. I understand that the Creator has a plan. However, I sometime wonder if we had known sooner; if things would have been different. It was at that time that I realized you can wait to long to address an ailment. But I think of Eddie daily with wonderful thoughts. And he left me with his beautiful family of four granddaughters and my daughter-in-law Clara Aburto.

Doctor Jasmine Martino, an inspiring herbalist who was informative and an inspiration while putting this book together. Dr. Cheryl J. Kincaide, was very enlightening. Lawrence Wilson, who was extremely helpful, James Ingram, who asked many questions, Linda Cunningham, RN who offered encouragement. Patricia Jones, who believed in me.

CONTENTS

VOLUME I OF 4

AIDS

*Aloe

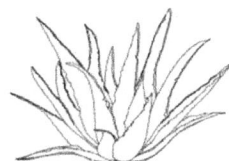

ALOE can be an excellent source for treating and combating the onset of AIDS. It buffers the HIV virus from entering cells, slowing the virus from moving throughout the body. Aloe cleanses the blood and the colon. It treats skin eruptions, abrasions, bedsores, and regulates the bowels. It helps with easing pain. Use the whole leaf of the Aloe. Wash and peel the Aloe leaves, place them in a juicer and drink it as it is, do not add sugar. Drink four to six ounces. Fresh Aloe leaves are best used for this ailment. It may be taken in capsules, if it is taken as a tea, use ¼ teaspoon of Aloe herb powder to one cup of boiling water. Aloe may be taken as often as you feel the need. For treating HIV/AIDS it may be taken once or twice a day, for two to ten days, or until desired results are reached. For some, two or three times a week will be beneficial.

Contains: calcium, iron, sodium, potassium, magnesium, lecithin, and zinc.

Amaranth

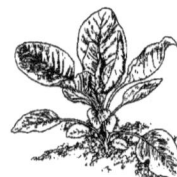

AMARANTH will be helpful for treating AIDS. It counters the emergence of herpes and it will help with the treatment of diarrhea. It treats hemorrhaging, and the spitting up of blood. It treats several viruses and helps to boost the immune system. Amaranth may be taken in capsules. If it is taken as a tea, use ½ teaspoon of Amaranth herb powder to one cup of boiling water. Amaranth may be taken as often as you feel the need. For AIDS it may be taken two or three times a day, or until desired results are reached. For some, three or four times a week can be helpful.

Contains: vitamin C, magnesium, potassium and niacin. Amaranth is very high in protein, iron, calcium, and has a high concentration of amino acid L-Lysine.

AIDS

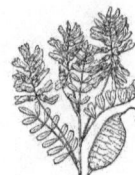

Astragalus

ASTRAGALUS is excellent for treating AIDS. It boosts the immune system and is good to take when you suffer chronic fatigue. It strengthens the T-cells and helps with chronic lesions. Astragalus helps to improve urine flow; urination will increase while using it. It helps to reduce blood pressure. It treats heart disease, improves circulation and treats uterine cancer. It may be taken in capsules. If it is taken as a tea, use ½ teaspoons of Astragalus herb powder to one cup of boiling water.

Contains: choline, betaine, and glucoronic acid.

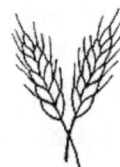

**Barley Juice Powder*

BARLEY JUICE POWDER can be great for treating AIDS. It is a booster for the immune system, which is vital to a person with AIDS. It builds the blood, purifies the blood, and treats fatigue, and anemia. Barley Juice Powder is an excellent treatment for cancer. It removes heavy metals and lead from the body. Barley Juice Powder may suppress the appetite. Fresh Barley leaves may be juiced for drinking. It may be taken in capsules. If it is taken as a tea, use ½ teaspoons of Barley Juice Powder to one cup of boiling water. Barley juice may be taken as often as you feel the need. For treating AIDS it may be taken once a day for two to seven days. For some, two or three times a week can be excellent.

Contains: vitamins B1, B12, C, potassium, and is high in iron and calcium.

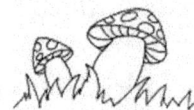

**Reish/Mushroom*

REISHI/MUSHROOM can be excellent for treating AIDS. It will inhibit replication of the HIV virus. It treats chronic fatigue, stimulates T-cells, and will boost the immune system. It relieves stress and has been known to lower cholesterol, and strengthen the heart. It helps to slow the progress of cancer, and helps to enhance longevity. It may be taken in capsules. If it is taken as a tea, use ¼ teaspoon of Reishi/Mushroom

AIDS

herb powder to one cup of boiling water. Reishi/Mushroom may be taken as often as you feel the need. For combating AIDS it may be taken once or twice a day, for two to ten days, or until desired results are reached. For some, two or three times a week can be beneficial.

*Pau D'Arco

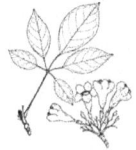

Pau D'Arco can be very beneficial for treating AIDS. It starts with purifying the blood and enhancing the immune system. It is known to increase red corpuscles. It has strong virus killing powers. It treats cancer, herpes and hepatitis. It helps to neutralize poisons in the liver. It can be very beneficial during chemotherapy use. It may be taken in capsules, if it is taken as a tea use ¼ teaspoon of Pau D'Arco herb powder to one cup of boiling water. Pau D'Arco may be taken as often as you feel the need. For AIDS it may be taken once or twice a day, for two to seven days, or until desired results are reached. For some, once or twice a week can be beneficial to build the red blood cells.

Contains: potassium, sodium, magnesium, manganese, selenium, zinc, and vitamins A, B complex, and C, and is very high in iron.

*Red Clover

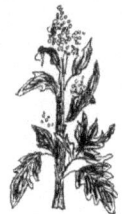

Red Clover can be an excellent choice for treating AIDS. It will boost the immune system. It gives a laxative effect on the system. It is a tonic and will calm the nerves and add energy. It can also be helpful for clearing mucus from the system. It can be great for treating the esophagus. It helps to prevent the spread of infection. It can be excellent to use as an external wash for boils and sores. Red Clover will stimulate the liver. It may be taken in capsules. If it is taken as a tea, use ¼ teaspoon of Red Clover herb powder to one cup of boiling water. Red Clover may be taken as often as you feel the need. For AIDS it may be taken once a day, for two to five days, or until desired results are reached. For some, once or twice a week can be beneficial.

Contains: vitamins A, B complex, calcium, sodium, nickel, manganese, and tin.

ALZHEIMER'S

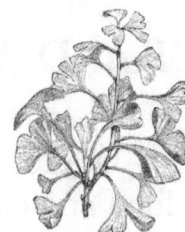

*Ginkgo

GINKGO is excellent for treating Alzheimer's. It offers alertness, treats depression, and mood swings. It treats senility, memory loss and it increases attention span. Ginkgo may be taken in capsules, if it is taken as a tea, use ¼ teaspoon of Ginkgo herb powder to one cup of boiling water. Ginkgo offers more benefits taken without sweetener. Ginkgo may be taken as often as you feel the need. For Alzheimer's disease it may be taken once or twice a day, for two to ten days, or until desired results are reached. For some, once or twice a week can be beneficial for two to three weeks.

Contains bioflavonoids.

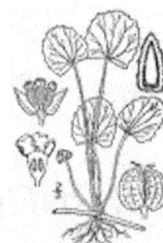

*Gotu Kola

GOTO KOLA can be excellent for treating Alzheimer's. It increases energy, treats memory loss, increases mental alertness, treats senility, and strengthens the heart. It also increases circulation to the brain and treats depression. Goto Kola is a diuretic. It may be taken in capsules, if it is taken as a tea, use ¼ teaspoon of Goto Kola herb powder to one cup of boiling water. Goto Kola may be taken as often as you feel the need. For Alzheimer's disease it may be taken once or twice a day, for two to ten days, or until desired results are reached. For some, two or three times a week can be beneficial for a few weeks.

Contains: vitamins A, G, and K, and it is high in magnesium.

ARTHRITIS

Alfalfa

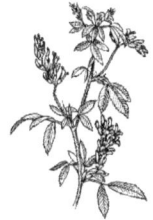

ALFALFA can be great for treating arthritis. It helps to remove inflammation in the joints, and reduces swelling. It also offers relief from pain, treats bursitis, gout, rheumatism, fatigue, acidity and asthma. It purifies the blood, and offers colon cancer prevention. It will enhance the immune system. Alfalfa may be taken in capsules. If it is taken as a tea, use ¼ teaspoon of Alfalfa herb powder to one cup of boiling water. Alfalfa may be taken as often as you feel the need, for chronic arthritis it may be taken two or three times a day for four to five days, or until desired results are reached, For some, once or twice a week can be beneficial.

Herbs for your blood type: Alfalfa is highly beneficial for people with blood type A. It is neutral for people with blood type B and AB. People with blood type O should avoid this herb it will cause excessive blood thinning for them.

Contains: vitamins A, B complex, D, E, K, iron, potassium, magnesium, protein, sodium, sulfur and phosphorus. Alfalfa is very high in calcium, chlorophyll, and vitamin B12.

Angelica

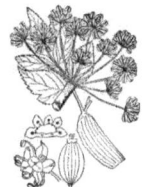

ANGELICA will assist with treating the pain of arthritis. It is a tonic and can be strengthening and invigorating to the system. Angelica also treats bronchial problems, colds, colic, exhaustion, heartburn, and rheumatism. Angelica will stimulate the appetite and will increase urination. **Angelica should be used with caution if you are a diabetic:** it will elevate sugar in the blood. **Do not take Angelica if you suffer excessive bleeding.** Do not use Angelica during pregnancy: it may

ARTHRITIS

HERBS:

induce a miscarriage. Angelica may be taken in capsules, if it is taken as a tea, use ¼ teaspoon of Angelica herb powder to one cup of boiling water. Angelica may be taken as often as you feel the need. For arthritis it may be taken once or twice a day, for two to five days, or until desired results are reached. For some, two or three times a week can be beneficial for prevention.

Contains: vitamins E, B 12, and calcium.

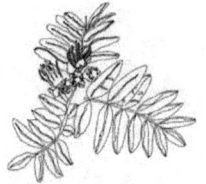

Astragalus

ASTRAGALUS will help with treating arthritis. It is also an anti-inflammatory that protects against chemical damage caused by chemotherapy. It also treats, uterine cancer, colds, and strengthens the digestive system; it treats liver problems, increases energy, and helps to normalize blood pressure. It strengthens the T-cells and helps with chronic lesions and AIDS. Urination will increase while using Astragalus. It may be taken in capsules. If it is taken as a tea, use ¼ teaspoons of Astragalus herb powder to one cup of boiling water. Astragalus may be taken as often as you feel the need. For arthritis it may be taken once or twice a day, for four to five days, or until desired results are reached. For some, once or twice a week can be helpful.

Contains: choline, betaine, and gluconic acid.

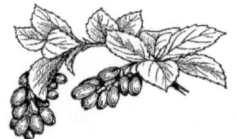

Barberry

BARBERRY will help to treat arthritis. It relieves inflammation in the joints. It also stimulates and soothes the muscles. It purifies the blood, treats diarrhea, and fevers. Barberry treats a sluggish gallbladder, indigestion, infections, jaundice, and liver conditions. It treats ulcers in the mouth, sore throat, syphilis and typhoid fever. **Barberry should not be used excessively it may cause depression.** Barberry may be taken in capsules, if it is taken as a tea use ¼ teaspoon of Barry herb powder to one cup of boiling water. Barberry may be taken as often as you feel the need. For arthritis it may be taken once or twice a day, for three to five days, or until desired

ARTHRITIS

results are reached. For some, once or twice a week can give results in a short period of time.

Contains: iron, manganese, phosphorus, and vitamin C.

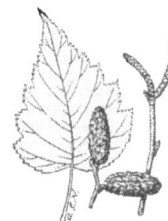

*Birch

BIRCH works great for relieving the pain of arthritis. It also treats rheumatism and bladder problems. It cleanses the blood, and treats cancer. Birch is a diuretic and a sedative. Birch can be taken at bedtime for insomnia. Birch may be taken in capsules, if it is taken as a tea, use ¼ teaspoon of Birch herb powder to one cup of boiling water. Birch may be taken as often as you feel the need. For arthritis it may be taken once or twice a day, for three to five days, or until desired results are reached. For some, once or twice a week will give results in a short period.

Contains: copper, sodium, calcium, iron, magnesium, potassium, silicon, vitamins A, B1, B2, C, and E

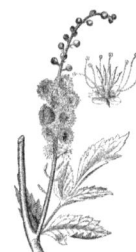

Black Cohosh

BLACK COHOSH will assist with the treatment of arthritis. It treats inflammation in the joints, rheumatism, and spinal meningitis. It also treats asthma, chronic bronchitis, and helps with childbirth. It's great for treating dropsy, epilepsy, and fevers. It reduces hot flashes, treats hysteria, malaria, and menstrual problems, and cleans the blood. **Black Cohosh is a sedative and should be used in small amounts or it can cause a headache.** It lowers the heart rate slightly but increases the pulse rate. **Black Cohosh will work to induce labor when pregnant.** Black Cohosh may be taken in capsules. When it is taken as a tea, use 1/8th teaspoon or less of Black Cohosh herb powder to one cup of boiling water. Black Cohosh may be taken as often as you feel the need. For arthritis it may be taken once a day for three to five

---

ARTHRITIS

---

days, or until desired results are reached. As a preventative once or twice a week for two to three weeks should give results.

Contains: calcium, potassium, iron, magnesium, manganese, niacin, phosphorus, selenium, silicon, sodium, sulphur, vitamins A, B1, B2, C, K, and F, and zinc.

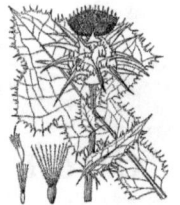

Blessed Thistle

BLESSED THISTLE can be useful for treating arthritis. It treats poor circulation, purifies the blood, stimulates brain activity, and it removes calcium deposits from the body in addition to treating, cancer, and depression. It is also great for treating digestive disorders, fevers, gas, and headaches. It treats angina, balances hormones, hysteria, and liver conditions. It strengthens the lungs and treats vaginal discharge. It may be taken in capsules. If it is taken as a tea, use ¼ teaspoon of Blessed Thistle herb to one cup of boiling water. Blessed Thistle may be taken as often as you feel the need. For arthritis it may be taken once or twice a day, for three to five days, or until desired results are reached. For some, once or twice a week can give results.

Contains: B complex, calcium, iron, manganese, and potassium.

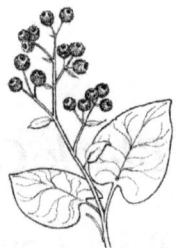

*Burdock

BURDOCK is great for treating chronic and advanced arthritis. It treats bursitis, rheumatism, and the sciatica nerve. It also cleans the blood, treats boils, cancer, constipation, and eczema, fluid retention, gout, itching, and kidney and liver problems. Burdock will increase urine flow. **An excessive amount of Burdock taken at once may cause vomiting.** Burdock may be taken in capsules. When it is taken as tea use ¼ teaspoon of Burdock herb powder to one cup of boiling water. Burdock may be taken as often as you feel the need. For arthritis it may be taken once or twice a day, for three to four days, or until desired results are reached. For some, once or twice a week will be beneficial.

ARTHRITIS

HERBS:

Herbs for your blood type: Burdock is highly beneficial for people with blood type A and AB. It is neutral for people with blood type B. People with blood type O should avoid this herb it will cause excessive blood thinning and excessive bleeding.

Contains: vitamins A, B complex, C, E, iron, zinc, and sulphur.

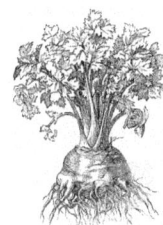

*Celery Root

CELERY ROOT can be great for relief from arthritis. It treats severe and crippling arthritis; gout, rheumatism, lumbago, cancer, and nervousness. It will produce a calming effect on the nervous system. It may be taken in capsules. If it is taken as a tea, use ¼ teaspoon of Celery herb powder to one cup of boiling water. Celery may be taken as often as you feel the need. For arthritis it may be taken once or twice a day, for three to seven days, or until desired results are reached. For some, two or three times a week can be beneficial.

Contains: potassium, sodium, calcium, vitamins A, B, and C, and is high in iron.

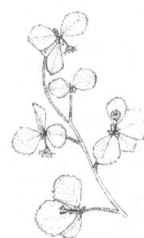

*Chaparral

CHAPARRAL will be excellent for treating arthritis. It reduces inflammation in the joints, treats rheumatism, it is also excellent for cancer, leukemia, skin diseases and tumors. It is cleansing to the lymph system and it is powerful for removing parasites. Chaparral may elevate blood pressure for some people when taken excessively. Chaparral may be taken in capsules, if it is taken as a tea use ¼ teaspoon of Chaparral herb powder to one cup of boiling water. Chaparral may be taken as often as you feel the need. For arthritis it may be taken once or twice a day, for three to five days, or until desired results are reached. For some, two or three times a week can be beneficial for prevention.

ARTHRITIS

Contains: sodium, potassium, aluminum, barium, chlorine, protein, silicon, and sulphur.

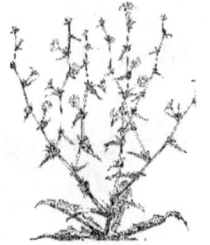

Chicory

CHICORY helps to relieve the pain of arthritis. It treats stiffness in the joints. Chicory will help to remove calcium deposits; it is a blood purifier, it treats inflammation in the system, and helps to remove excessive mucus in the body. It will help with the pain relief. It may be taken in capsules, if it is taken as a tea, use ¼ teaspoon of Chicory herb powder to one cup of boiling water. Chicory may be taken as often as you feel the need. For arthritis it may be taken once or twice a day, for three to six days, or until desired results are reached. For some, once or twice a week can be beneficial.

Contains: a high amount of vitamins A, B, C, K, and P.

Chlorella

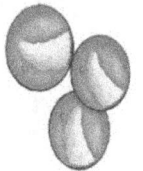

CHLORELLA can be useful for treating arthritis. It also treats allergies, and cancerous growths. It lowers blood pressure and cholesterol. It treats liver toxicity. It will be useful for removing heavy metals from the body such as lead, mercury and copper. It helps to protect against the effects of ultraviolet radiation. It may be taken in capsules, if it is taken as a tea, use ¼ teaspoon of chlorella herb powder to one cup of boiling water. Chlorella may be taken as often as you feel the need. For arthritis it may be taken once a day for three to five days, or until desired results are reached. For some, once or twice a week can be helpful.

Contains: vitamins B1, B2, B6, B12, C, and E. Chlorella is high in chlorophyll, and many minerals.

ARTHRITIS

Cinnamon

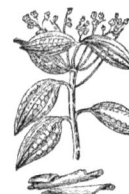

CINNAMON can be helpful for reducing the discomfort of arthritis. **Women should avoid Cinnamon during pregnancy. Men with prostate problems should avoid cinnamon. Diabetics should consult a health care provider before taking Cinnamon.** Some herbalists say it will increase insulin activity. Cinnamon may be used as a spice in the kitchen. It may be taken in capsules. If it is taken as a tea, use ¼ teaspoon of Cinnamon herb powder to one cup of boiling water. Cinnamon may be taken as often as you feel the need. For arthritis it may be taken two or three times a day for two to five days, or until desired results are reached. For some, once a week can be helpful.

Herbs for your blood type: Cinnamon is neutral for people with blood type A and blood type AB. People with blood type O and blood type B should avoid this herb.

Contains calcium, chromium, copper, iodine, manganese, potassium, zinc, tannins, vitamins A, B, and C.

*Dandelion

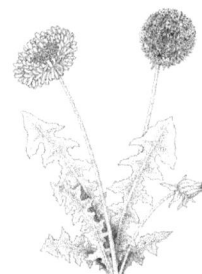

DANDELION can be excellent for treating arthritis. It reduces stiffness in the joints, treats infections, and offers endurance. It purifies the blood, is excellent for treating skin disease, anemia, and asthma. Dandelion is a diuretic. **Dandelion may elevate blood pressure for some people when taken excessively.** Dandelion may be taken in capsules, if it is taken as a tea, use ¼ teaspoon of Dandelion herb powder to one cup of boiling water. Dandelion may be taken as often as you feel the need. For arthritis it may be taken once or twice a day, for three to five days, or until desired results are reached. For some, once or twice a week can be beneficial.

Herbs for your blood type: Dandelion is highly beneficial for people with blood type O. It is neutral for people with blood type A, B, and AB.

Contains calcium, vitamins A, B, C, and E, sodium, potassium, iron, nickel, tin, copper magnesium, manganese, sulphur, and zinc.

ARTHRITIS

Devil's Claw

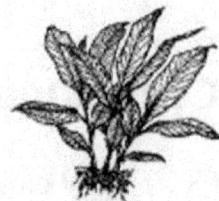

DEVIL'S CLAW treats rheumatoid arthritis. It reduces inflammation in the joints and strengthens the whole system while it works. It treats neuralgia and gout. It also removes toxic impurities from the body, treats Arteriosclerosis; bladder problems, cholesterol, diabetes, headaches, kidney, liver diseases, and stomach disorders. Devil's Claw may be taken in capsules. If it is taken as a tea, use ¼ teaspoon of Devil's Claw herb powder to one cup of boiling water. Devil's Claw may be taken as often as you feel the need. For arthritis it may be taken once or twice a day, for two to ten days, or until desired results are reached. For some, once or twice a year will help with prevention.

Contains calcium, iron, magnesium, manganese, phosphorus, potassium, protein, selenium, silicon, sodium, vitamins A and C, and zinc.

Dong Quai

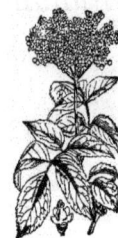

DONG QUAI offers assistance for treating arthritis. It increases circulation, treats anemia, purifies the blood, and treats cancer. It also treats female problems, prolapsed uterus, migraine headaches, and muscle spasms. It can be great for treating nervousness and it is excellent for treating hot flashes, they just seem to disappear. Dong Quai may be taken in capsules. If it is taken as tea, use ¼ teaspoon of Dong Quai herb powder to one cup of boiling water. Dong Quai may be taken as often as you feel the need. For arthritis it may be taken once or twice a day, for two to five days, or until desired results are reached. For some, once or twice a week will be beneficial.

Herbs for your blood type: Dong Quai is neutral for people with blood type O, A, B and AB.

Contains vitamins A, B12, and E, and is very high in iron.

ARTHRITIS

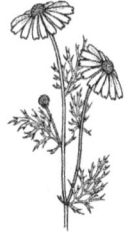

*Feverfew

FEVERFEW will be excellent for treating arthritis. It will reduce inflammation in the joints. It treats muscle tension, tinnitus, and vertigo. It can also be excellent for treating hay fever, and sinus headaches. Feverfew will do wonders for migraine headaches. Feverfew will promote menstruation. It may be taken in capsules. If it is taken as a tea, use ¼ teaspoon of Feverfew herb powder to one cup of boiling water. Feverfew may be taken as often as you feel the need. For arthritis it may be taken once or twice days for four to five days, or until desired results are reached. For some, once or twice a week can be beneficial.

Feverfew may elevate blood pressure for some people when used excessively. If it must be taken, use only a pinch of Feverfew in combination with other herbs.

Contains vitamins A and C, iron, niacin, potassium, selenium, sodium, and zinc.

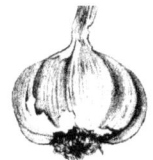

*Garlic

GARLIC can be very effective in treating arthritis. It improves circulation, and helps to regulate blood pressure. It also treats cancer, cholera, lungs, and detoxifies the liver. Garlic also treats prostate problems, and yeast infections. **Garlic may elevate blood pressure for some people when taken excessively.** It may be taken in capsules. If it is taken as a tea, use ¼ teaspoon of Garlic herb powder to one cup of boiling water. Garlic may be taken as often as you feel the need. For arthritis it may be taken two or three times a day for two to seven days, or until desired results are reached. For some, two or three times a week can helpful.

Herbs for your blood type: Garlic is highly beneficial for people with blood type A and AB. It is neutral for people with blood type O and B.

Contains sodium, sulphur, calcium, copper, vitamin B1, iron, and is high in potassium, zinc selenium, and vitamins A and C.

ARTHRITIS

Ginkgo

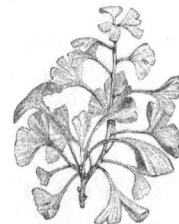

GINKGO offers relief from arthritis. It stimulates circulation, treats Alzheimer's disease, strokes, memory loss, and hearing. It can be strengthening to the vascular system and it helps to decrease blood clots. It may be taken in capsules. If it is taken as a tea, use ¼ teaspoon of Ginkgo herb powder to one cup of boiling water. Ginkgo may be taken as often as you feel the need. For arthritis it may be taken once or twice a day, for three to four days, or until desired results are reached. For some, once or twice a week can be beneficial.

Contains bioflavonoids.

Golden Rod

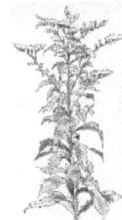

GOLDEN ROD will help to treat chronic and acute arthritis. It also helps with treating diarrhea, gas, kidney and urinary problems. It is a diuretic. Golden Rod may be taken in capsules. If it is taken as tea, use ¼ teaspoon of Golden Rod herb powder to one cup of boiling water. Golden Rod may be taken as often as you feel the need. For arthritis it may be taken once or twice a day, for three to five days, or until desired results are reached. For some, once or twice a week for two weeks will be beneficial.

Horseradish

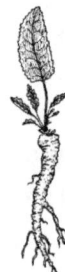

HORSERADISH can be used as a balm for arthritis. It treats stiffness and arthritis pain. Mix Horseradish with olive oil and make a paste and rub on the affected area several times a day.

ARTHRITIS

HERBS:

*Horsetail

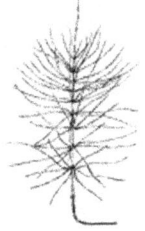

HORSETAIL is excellent for treating arthritis. It increases circulation. It also great for treating diabetes, hair loss, kidney stones, and weak and brittle nails. Horsetail treats parasites, decreases bleeding, and keeps calcium in the body. It will increase urination during use. **Horsetail may elevate blood pressure for some people when taken excessively.** Horsetail may be taken in capsules. If it is taken as a tea, use ¼ teaspoon of Horsetail herb powder to one cup of boiling water. Horsetail may be taken as often as you feel the need. For arthritis it may be taken once or twice a day, for three to five days, or until desired results are reached. For some once or twice a week can be helpful.

Contains sodium, iron, iodine, copper, vitamin E, selenium, and a high content of silicon.

Hydrangea

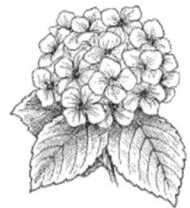

HYDRANGEA will help to give relief from chronic arthritis. It also treats rheumatism, gout, and stones in the bladder. It treats bladder infections, gallstones, gonorrhea, kidney stones and urinary problems. **Hydrangea may elevate blood pressure for some, people when taken excessively. People with high blood pressure should not use Hydrangea herb more then once a week.** Hydrangea may be taken in capsules, if it is taken as a tea, use ¼ teaspoon of Hydrangea herb powder to one cup of boiling water. Hydrangea may be taken as often as you feel the need. For treating arthritis it may be taken once or twice a day, for three to five days, or until desired results are reached. For some, once or twice a week can be helpful.

Contains sodium, sulphur, calcium, iron, potassium, and magnesium.

ARTHRITIS

HERBS:

Juniper

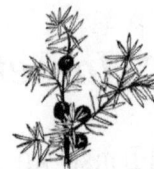

JUNIPER is helpful for the prevention of arthritis. It gives a healing effect to the entire system. It also treats infections, colds, diabetes, dropsy, and kidney problems. It treats the pancreas and prostate gland. Do not use Juniper if there is kidney disease, it may over stimulate the kidneys. Pregnant women should not take Juniper. Juniper may be taken in capsules. If it is taken as a tea, use ¼ teaspoon of Juniper to one cup of boiling water. Juniper may be taken as often as you feel the need. For arthritis it may be taken once or twice a day, for three to five days, or until desired results are reached. For some, once or twice a week can be helpful.

Contains sulphur, copper, a small amount of aluminum, and a high amount of vitamin C.

*Kelp

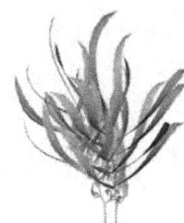

KELP can be especially useful for treating arthritis. It cleans the arteries, removes lead from the body and enhances the immune system. Kelp also treats colitis, diabetes, and eczema. It will increase energy and suppress the appetite. Kelp is very high in minerals, and promotes healthy hair growth. It may be taken in capsules. If it is taken as a tea, use ¼ teaspoon of Kelp herb powder to one cup of boiling water. Kelp may be taken as often as you feel the need. For treating arthritis it may be taken once or twice a day, for three to seven days, or until desired results are reached. For some, once or twice a week can be beneficial.

Contains calcium, chlorine, sulphur, silicon, zinc, manganese, aluminum, potassium, copper, nickel, iron, silver, phosphorus, vanadium, B complex, vitamins A, C, E, and K, and a very high content of iodine and minerals.

ARTHRITIS

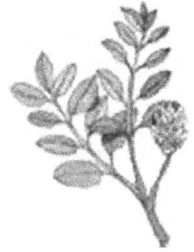

Licorice

LICORICE stimulates the joints in the body while treating arthritis. It offers relief from the pain. It also treats Addison's disease, increases energy; treats weight loss, and gastrointestinal problems. It may be taken in capsules. If it is taken as a tea, use ¼ teaspoon Licorice herb powder to one cup of boiling water. Licorice may be taken as often as you feel the need. For treating arthritis it may be taken once or twice a day, for four to six days, or until desired results are reached. For some, two or three times a week will offer desired results.

Herbs for your blood type: Licorice is highly beneficial for people with blood type B and AB. It is neutral for people with blood type O and A.

Contains niacin, lecithin, iodine, chromium, zinc, and vitamins E and B complex.

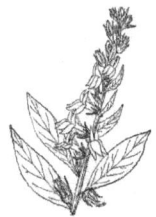

*Lobelia

LOBELIA has an excellent healing effect on arthritis. It also treats pain, infections, acute asthma attacks, bronchitis, chicken pox, emphysema, epilepsy, fevers, migraine headaches, pneumonia and seizures. Lobelia increases urine flow. It may be taken in capsules. If it is taken as a tea, add ¼ teaspoon of Lobelia herb powder to one cup of boiling water. Lobelia may be taken as often as you feel the need. For arthritis it may be taken once a day for two to five days, or until desired results are reached. For some, two or three times a week can offer desired results.

Contains iron, copper, sodium, sulphur, cobalt, lead, and selenium.
LOTS OF WATER SHOULD BE TAKEN WITH LOBELIA.

ARTHRITIS

Myrrh

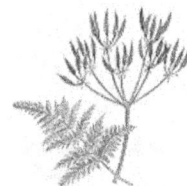

MYRRH will assist with treating arthritis. It is a stimulant that brings order to the entire system. It also treats pain, asthma, bronchitis, and colds, it freshens the breath and cleanses the stomach. Myrrh has antiseptic properties and it may be used in place of Golden Seal. Myrrh will stimulate and promote menstruation. Myrrh may elevate blood pressure for some people when taken excessively. **Myrrh may be taken in capsules.** If it is taken as a tea, use ¼ teaspoon of Myrrh herb powder to one cup of boiling water. Myrrh may be taken as often as you feel the need. For arthritis it may be taken once or twice a day, for three to seven days, or until desired results are reached. For some, once or twice a week can be beneficial.

Contains potassium, sodium, chlorine, silicon, and zinc.

*Oatstraw

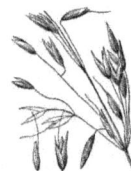

OATSTRAW can be very effective for the relief of arthritis. It also strengthens the heart, and treats indigestion, insomnia, nervous problems, and the urinary organs. If one is recovering from an illness, or drug withdrawals, this herb will help with recovery. It stimulates the appetite and helps to lower blood pressure and cholesterol. Oatstraw can be helpful for treating thyroid and estrogen deficiency. Oatstraw is best taken at bedtime. Oatstraw may be taken in capsules. If it is taken as a tea, use ¼ teaspoon of Oatstraw herb powder to one cup of boiling water. Oatstraw may be taken as often as you feel the need. For chronic arthritis it may be taken once or twice a day, for three to five days, or until desired results are reached. For some once or twice a week may be beneficial

Contains: vitamins A, B1, B2, and E, and is high in calcium and silicon.

ARTHRITIS

Oregon Grape

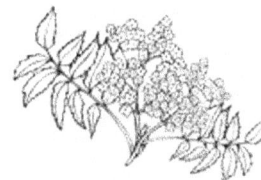

OREGON GRAPE will assist with treating rheumatoid arthritis. It is a good herb to start with for treating arthritis. It will strengthen the immune system and combat cancer. Oregon Grape increases the appetite; it purifies the blood, treats eczema, jaundice, and infections, cleans the liver, and helps with constipation. Oregon Grape will stimulate the thyroid functions. It may be taken in capsules. If it is taken as a tea, use ¼ teaspoon of Oregon Grape herb powder, to one cup of boiling water. Oregon Grape may be taken as often as you feel the need. For arthritis it may be taken once or twice a day, for three to five days, or until desired results are reached. For some, once or twice a week will be helpful for desired results.

Contains: sodium, zinc, manganese, copper, and silicon.

Parsley

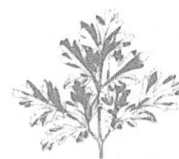

PARSLEY will help to treat arthritis. It stimulates circulation and increases the appetite. Parsley is a diuretic and will help when urination is painful. Parsley should be used in moderation during pregnancy: it will induce labor pains. It is also beneficial for mother's to use after birth, it will dry up mother's milk during the weaning period. It may be taken in capsules, if it is taken as a tea use ¼ teaspoon of Parsley herb powder to one cup of boiling water. Parsley may be taken as often as you feel the need. For arthritis it may be taken once or twice a day, for two to seven days, or until desired results are reached. For some, once or twice a week can be helpful for desired results.

Herbs for your blood type: Parsley is highly beneficial for people with blood type O and B. It is neutral for people with blood type A and AB.

Contains: vitamins A, B and C, chlorophyll, iron, potassium, calcium, cobalt, copper, riboflavin, silicon sodium, sulphur, and thiamine.

ARTHRITIS

HERBS:

*Pau D'Arco

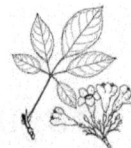

PAU D'ARCO is excellent for relieving the pain of arthritis. It also offers energy and has great cancer fighting abilities; it treats AIDS, acting as a blood purifier. It treats diabetes, eczema, Hodgkin's disease, leukemia, liver conditions, and yeast infections. It may be taken in capsules. If it is taken as a tea, use ¼ teaspoon of Pau D'Arco to one cup of boiling water. Pau D'Arco may be taken as often as you feel the need. For arthritis it may be taken once or twice a day, for three to five days, or until desired results are reached. For some, once or twice a week can be helpful.

Contains: potassium, sodium, magnesium, manganese, selenium, and zinc. Vitamins A, B complex, and C, and is very high in iron

*Pine Tree Bark

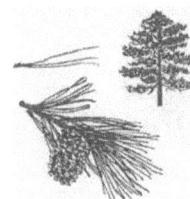

PINE TREE BARK is among the best herbs for treating arthritis. It will reduce inflammation in the lymphatic system, and improve circulation in the blood. It can remove heavy metals, such as copper from the blood. It helps to treat cancer, brain dysfunction, heart disease and stress. Pine Tree Bark may be taken in capsules. If it is taken as a tea, use ¼ teaspoon of Pine Tree Bark herb powder to one cup of boiling water. Pine Tree Bark may be taken as often as you feel the need. For arthritis it may be taken once or twice a day, for two to four days, or until desired results are reached. For some, once or twice a week can be beneficial.

Contains: bioflavonoids and vitamin C.

ARTHRITIS

HERBS:

Prickly Ash

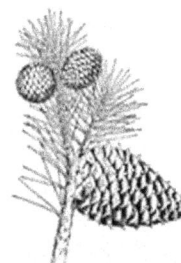

PRICKLY ASH works well for treating arthritis. It treats common complaints associated with arthritis. It will restore circulation to the body, help with treating joint problems, increase blood circulation, and help with leg cramps. Prickly Ash will increase the flow of saliva in the mouth. It can be applied externally as a balm to aide in direct relief of arthritis pain, while it is taken internally. It warms cold hands, cold feet, and cold legs. It may cause some people to become more sensitive to sunlight and burn more easily. It helps to treat yeast growth and gonorrhea. Prickly Ash may be taken in capsules. If it is taken as a tea, use ¼ teaspoon of prickly ash herb powder to one cup of boiling water. Prickly Ash may be taken as often as you feel the need. For arthritis it may be taken once or twice a day, for three to five days, or until desired results are reached. For some, two or three times a week can give desired results.

Contains tannins.

Red Clover

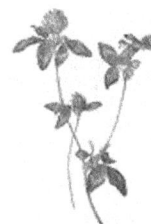

RED CLOVER can be useful for treating rheumatoid arthritis. It also helps to treat gout, and remove toxins from the body. It quiets the nerves and fights off cancer. Red Clover helps to strengthen the bladder, purifies the blood, and treats leukemia and liver problems. It may be taken in capsules, if it is taken as a tea, use ¼ teaspoon of Red Clover herb powder to one cup of boiling water. Red Clover may be taken as often as you feel the need. For arthritis it may be taken once or twice a day, for two to three days, or until desired results are reached.

Contains: vitamins A, B complex, calcium, sodium, nickel, manganese, tin, and is high in iron and calcium.

ARTHRITIS

HERBS:

Safflower

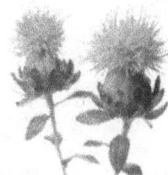

SAFFLOWER will help with relief from arthritis. It treats the pain; it treats gout, heartburn, hysteria, jaundice, and liver problems. It stimulates the appetite, and treats digestive disorders. Safflower increases perspiration, and the flow of urine. It stimulates the pancreas, clears phlegm from the lungs and will temporarily increase production of insulin. It may be taken in capsules. If it is taken as a tea, use 1/8th teaspoon of safflower herb powder to one cup of boiling water. Safflower may be taken as often as you feel the need. For treating arthritis it may be taken once a day, for two or three days, or until desired results are reached. For some once or twice a week can be helpful.

Contains vitamin K.

Saffron

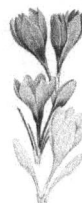

SAFFRON can offer effective results for relieving arthritis. It treats the discomfort of arthritis, and has anti-inflammatory abilities, treats rheumatism, gout, and acid-burning digestive disorders. It is best known for treating the gallbladder, liver, and scarlet fever. It may be taken in capsules. If it is taken as a tea, use ¼ teaspoon of Saffron herb powder to one cup of boiling water. Saffron may be taken as often as you feel the need. For arthritis it may be taken once or twice a day, for two to five days, or until desired results are reached. For some, once a week for two or three weeks can be helpful for prevention.

Contains: sodium, calcium, potassium, and vitamins A and B 12.

ARTHRITIS

HERBS:

Uva Ursi

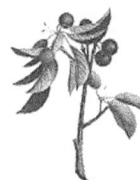

Uva Ursi can be effective for treating arthritis. It removes inflammation from anywhere in the body. It is excellent for treating Bright's disease, diabetes, gonorrhea; kidney infections and chronic urethritis. Begin by using a small amount of Uva Ursi and increase the amount as necessary. Uva Ursi increases the flow of urine and acts as a disinfectant. Uva Ursi will turn the urine a dark green, do not panic it is normal. **Large quantities of this herb should not be used during pregnancy it maybe harmful to the developing fetus.** Uva Ursi may be taken in capsules. If it is taken as a tea, use ¼ teaspoon of Uva Ursi to one cup of boiling water. Uva Ursi may be taken as often as you feel the need. For arthritis it may be taken once a day for three to seven days, or until desired results are reached. For some, two or three times a week can be helpful for achieving relief.

Contains: iron, manganese, trace minerals, and vitamin A.

Valerian

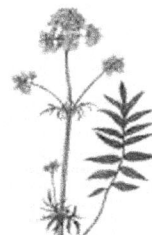

Valerian will assist with relieving arthritis. It treats pain and also treats after birth pains. It is excellent for treating hysteria, exhaustion and nervous breakdowns. It can be helpful to the rehabilitation of an addict. It acts as a sedative when taken. It helps to increase low concentration of sugar in the blood. **Valerian should not be taken for a long period of time it will cause mental depression. Do not give Valerian to children under age twelve.** Valerian has its own unique odor, similar to dirty socks. It may be taken in capsules. If it is taken as a tea, use ¼ teaspoon of Valerian herb powder to one cup of boiling water. Valerian may be taken as often as you feel the need. For treating arthritis it may be taken once a day for three to five days, or, until desired results are reached.

Herbs for your blood type: Valerian is highly beneficial for people with blood type A. It is neutral with people of blood type O, B and AB.

Contains: vitamins A and C, iron, sodium, potassium, niacin, calcium, magnesium, manganese, silicon, and selenium.

ARTHRITIS

HERBS:

*Wild Yam

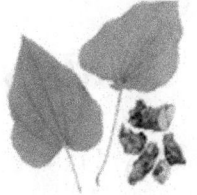

WILD YAM works great for treating acute arthritis. It can also be used to treat rheumatoid arthritis, relieve stiffness in the joints, treat muscle spasms, and general pain. Wild Yam will increase energy. It also treats Addison's disease, asthma, gas, and liver problems. Wild Yam will promote perspiration. It assists with weight loss, and gastrointestinal problems. Wild Yam may be taken in capsules. If it is taken as a tea, use ¼ teaspoon of Wild Yam herb powder to one cup of boiling water. Wild Yam may be taken as often as you feel the need. For chronic arthritis it may be taken once or twice, a day for three to five days, or until desired results are reached. For some, once a week can be beneficial

Yellow Dock

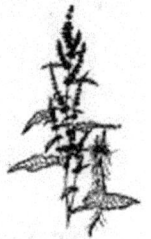

YELLOW DOCK can be helpful with treating arthritis. It treats rheumatism, scurvy, and blood disorders. It is a blood cleanser and a terrific tonic for the system. It also cleans the lymphatic system, treats cancer and infectious tumors. Yellow Dock may be taken in capsules. If it is taken as a tea, use ¼ teaspoon of Yellow Dock herb powder to one cup of boiling water. Yellow Dock may be taken as often as you feel the need. For arthritis it may be taken once or twice a day, for three to seven days, or until desired results are reached. For some once or twice a week can be beneficial in a short period.

Herbs for your blood type: Yellow Dock is neutral for people with blood type B and AB. People with blood type O, and A should avoid this herb.

Contains: vitamins A, C, and nickel, and is very high in iron.

ASTHMA

*Alfalfa

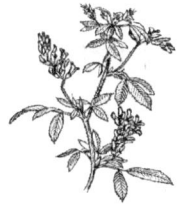

ALFALFA can be excellent for treating asthma. It has many functions for the system but one of its main functions is treating asthma. It treats fatigue, gout, acidity, allergies, and arthritis. It helps to prevent colon cancer when taken over a period of time. It treats nausea and chronic weakness. Alfalfa may be taken in capsules. If it is taken as a tea, use ¼ teaspoon of Alfalfa herb powder to one cup of boiling water. Alfalfa may be taken as often as you feel the need. For asthma it may be taken two or three times a day for three to five days, or until desired results are reached. For some, once or twice a week can be beneficial for prevention.

Herbs for your blood type: Alfalfa is highly beneficial for people with blood type A. It is neutral for people with blood type B and AB. People with blood type O should avoid this herb it will cause excessive blood thinning for them.

Contains: vitamins A, B complex, D, E, and K, iron, potassium, magnesium, protein, sodium, sulfur, and phosphorus, and is very high in calcium, chlorophyll, and vitamin B12.

Aloe

ALOE can be beneficial for treating asthma. There are a variety of Aloe plants and they are all very therapeutic and will boost the immune system and eliminate toxins from the body. It also treats acne, allergies, bedsores, burns, scalds, eczema, and wounds. Aloe may be taken in capsules, if it is taken as a tea, use ¼ teaspoon of Aloe herb powder to one cup of boiling water. Aloe may be taken as often as you feel the need. For asthma it may be taken once or twice a day, for three to five

ASTHMA

days, or until desired results are reached. For some, once or twice a week can be beneficial.

Herbs for your blood type: Aloe is highly beneficial for people with blood type A. People with blood type O, B, or AB should avoid Aloe.

Contains: calcium, iron, sodium, potassium, magnesium, lecithin, and zinc.

Barley Juice

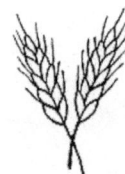

BARLEY JUICE will be helpful in relieving asthma. It treats lung problems, boosts the immune system, treats cancer, and removes metal poisoning. It purifies the blood and helps to reduce cholesterol. It can be taken in capsules, if it is taken as a tea, add ¼ teaspoon of Barley Juice herb powder to one cup of boiling water. Barley Juice may be taken as often as you feel the need. For asthma it may be taken once or twice a day, for four or five days, or until desired results are reached. For some, once or twice a week can be beneficial.

Contains: vitamins B1, B12, and C, potassium, iron, and is high in calcium.

*Bayberry

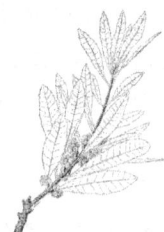

BAYBERRY can be very beneficial for the relief of asthma. It removes mucus from the lungs. Bayberry is a tonic that offers vitality to the body. It helps to clear the respiratory tract. It is also excellent to use as a douche for vaginal bleeding. It may be taken in capsules. If it is taken as a tea, use ¼ teaspoon of Bayberry herb powder to one cup of boiling water. Bayberry may be taken as often as you feel the need. For asthma it may be taken once or twice daily or as needed for relief. For some, two or three times a week can be beneficial.

Contains: potassium, sodium, niacin, calcium, magnesium, manganese, silicon, zinc, and vitamins B1, B2, and C.

ASTHMA

HERBS:

*Bee's Royal Jelly

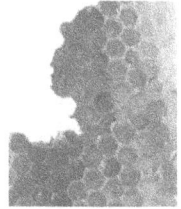

BEE'S ROYAL JELLY is an excellent herb for treating asthma. It offers energy, increases the immune system, offers longevity, and treats prostate problems. It helps to reduce cholesterol, and helps to reduce hazardous plaque out of blood vessels. Bee's Royal Jelly will promote sleep. It may be taken in capsules. If it is taken as a tea, use ¼ teaspoon of Bee's Royal Jelly herb powder to one cup of boiling water. Bee's Royal Jelly may be taken as often as you feel the need. For asthma it may be taken once or twice a day, for four to five days, or until desired results are reached. For some, once or twice a week can be beneficial. It is best taken at bedtime.

Contains: minerals, and is high in all of the B vitamins.

*Black Cohosh

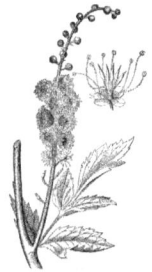

BLACK COHOSH is an excellent remedy for asthma. It is excellent for treating the lungs, as well as convulsions, diarrhea, epilepsy, spinal meningitis, and St.Vitus' Dance (Chorea). **Black Cohosh should be used in small amounts or it can cause a headache.** It lowers the heart rate slightly but increases the pulse rate. It reduces hot flashes and it is a sedative. **Black Cohosh will induce labor when pregnant.** Black Cohosh can be taken in capsules. If it is taken as a tea, use 1/8th teaspoon of Black Cohosh or less to one cup of boiling water. Black Cohosh may be taken as often as you feel the need. For asthma it may be taken once a day for three to four days, or until desired results are reached. For some, once a week can be helpful. Black Cohosh should be used in small amounts or it can cause a headache when taken excessively.

Contains: calcium, potassium, iron, magnesium, manganese, niacin, phosphorus, selenium, silicon, sodium, sulphur, vitamins A, B1, B2, C, K, and F, and zinc.

ASTHMA

Black Walnut

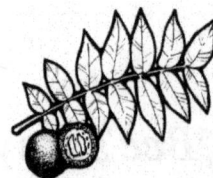

BLACK WALNUT can be effective for relief of asthma. It will also remove parasites from the body. It treats abscesses, acne, cancer, and herpes. It treats infections, lupus, tuberculosis and urinary problems. It lowers the thyroid function and it gives a laxative effect when used. It is very effective for treating bad blood. It has high organic iodine content. Black Walnut can be taken in capsules. If it is taken as a tea, use ¼ teaspoon of Black Walnut herb powder to one cup of boiling water. Black Walnut may be taken as often as you feel the need. For asthma it may be taken once or twice a day, for two to five days, or until desired results are reached. For some, once or twice a week can be beneficial.

Contains: magnesium, potassium, iron, calcium, and B15.

*Blue Vervain

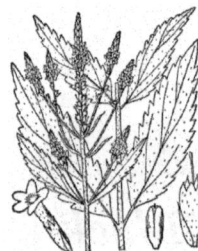

BLUE VERVAIN can be excellent for treating asthma. It clears the lungs, and soothes the upper respiratory system. It helps to stop the wheezing. It will calm the coughing that sometimes affects asthma suffers. Blue Vervain gives a calm and tranquilizing effect. Using large amounts of this herb at once may cause vomiting. It helps to expel waste from the system. It is a pleasant tasting herb and it may be taken in capsules. If it is taken as a tea, use ¼ teaspoon of Blue Vervain herb powder to one cup of boiling water.

Blue Vervain may be taken as often as you feel the need. For asthma it may be taken once or twice daily as needed for relief. For some, once or twice a week can be beneficial.

Contains: vitamin C, calcium, manganese, and vitamin E.

ASTHMA

Bugleweed

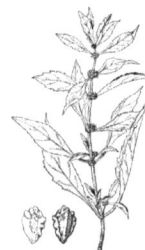

BUGLEWEED will assist with relief for asthma. It reduces mucus from the body and eliminates coughs. Bugleweed lowers the pulse and stabilizes an irregular heartbeat. It calms the nerves and the heart. Pregnant and nursing women should not use Bugleweed. Bugleweed may be taken in capsules. If it is taken as a tea, use ¼ teaspoon of Bugleweed herb powder to one cup of boiling water. Bugleweed may be taken as often as you feel the need. For some it may be taken once or twice a day, for two to five days, or until you receive the desired results. For some, once or twice a week can be beneficial.

Capsicum/Cayenne

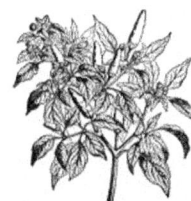

CAPSICUM/CAYENNE will help with the relief of asthma. It will remove fluid from the lungs. Capsicum/Cayenne stimulates circulation and increases perspiration. It has a hot peppery taste and can be used with other herbs. It may be taken in capsules. When it is taken as a tea use 1/8th teaspoon, or less, of Capsicum/Cayenne herb powder to one cup of boiling water. Capsicum/Cayenne may be taken as often as you feel the need. For asthma it may be taken once or twice a day until desired results are reached. For some, once or twice a week will be helpful.

Herbs for your blood type: Capsicum/Cayenne is highly beneficial for people with blood type O. It is neutral for people with blood B and AB. People with blood type A should avoid this herb.

Contains: vitamins A and C, magnesium, sulphur, and it is very high in iron, potassium, and calcium.

ASTHMA

HERBS:

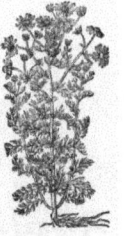

Chamomile

CHAMOMILE will assist with treating asthma. It is calming and soothing to the nerves, which is helpful for asthma sufferers. It helps to relax and reduce upset stomach problems. It stimulates the appetite, and it treats poor circulation, drug addictions, and fever. It may be taken in capsules, if it taken as a tea, use ¼ teaspoon of Chamomile herb powder to one cup of boiling water. Chamomile may be taken as often as you feel the need. For asthma it may be taken once or twice a day, for two to five days, or until desired results are reached. For some, once or twice a week can be helpful.

Herbs for your blood type: Chamomile is highly beneficial for people with blood type A and AB. It is neutral for people with blood type O, and B.

Contains: potassium, calcium, iron, manganese, vitamin A, and zinc.

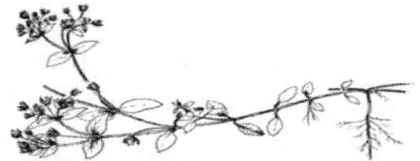

Chickweed

CHICKWEED will assist with treating asthma. It gives relief to the lungs and eliminates coughs. Chickweed also treats acne, allergies, and it purifies the blood. It lowers cholesterol and suppresses the appetite. Chickweed may elevate blood pressure for some people when taken excessively. It may be taken in capsules, if it is taken as a tea, use ¼ teaspoon of Chickweed herb powder to one cup of boiling water. Chickweed may be taken as often as you feel the need. For asthma it may be taken once or twice a day, for three to four days, or until desired results are reached. For some, once or twice a week can assist with relief.

Herbs for your Blood type: Chickweed is highly beneficial for people with blood type O. It is neutral for people with blood type A, B, and AB.

Contains: vitamins D, B complex, sodium, zinc, and is high in iron, vitamin C, minerals, calcium, and copper.

ASTHMA

HERBS:

Cinnamon

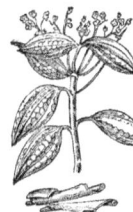

CINNAMON can be helpful for treating asthma. It has a calming effect on the body. It also improves the digestion system. It offers treatment for abdominal spasms, diarrhea, gas, and cancer. Pregnant women should avoid Cinnamon during pregnancy. Men with prostate problems should avoid cinnamon. Diabetics should consult a health care provider before taking Cinnamon. Some herbalists say it will increase insulin activity. Cinnamon may be used as a spice in the kitchen. It may be taken in capsules, if it is taken as a tea, use ¼ teaspoon of cinnamon herb powder to one cup of boiling water. Cinnamon may be taken as often as you feel the need. For asthma it may be taken once or twice a day, for three or four days, or until desired results are reached. For some, once or twice a week can be helpful until desired results are reached.

Herbs for your Blood type: Cinnamon is neutral for people with blood type A and blood type AB. People with blood type O and blood type B should avoid this herb.

Contains: calcium, chromium, copper, iodine, manganese, potassium, zinc, tannins, B-vitamins, and vitamins A and C.

*Coltsfoot

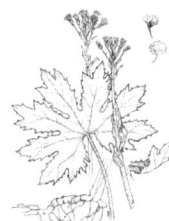

COLTSFOOT can be an excellent remedy for treating asthma. It has been known to sedate the wheezing and the coughs. It clears mucus from the lungs. Some people have been known to smoke Coltsfoot for asthma relief. It may be taken in capsules. It is a pleasant tasting herb. If it is taken as a tea, use ¼ teaspoon of Coltsfoot herb powder to one cup of boiling water. Coltsfoot may be taken as often as you feel the need. For chronic asthma problems it may be taken once or twice a day, for three to four days, or until desired results are achieved. For some, once or twice a week can be beneficial. Coltsfoot may elevate blood pressure for some people when taken excessively.

Herbs for your Blood type: Coltsfoot is highly beneficial for people with blood type A. People with blood type O, B and AB should avoid this herb.

ASTHMA

HERBS:

Contains: a rich amount of vitamins A and C; it has calcium, potassium, manganese, copper, zinc; vitamins P, B12, and B6.

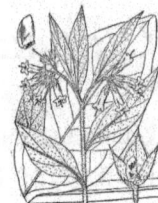

*Comfrey

COMFREY is excellent for treating asthma. It treats the respiratory system and moistens the lungs. Asthma sufferers should keep this herb on hand. It treats allergies, anemia, bladder problems, and it cleans the blood. It treats cancer, emphysema, pneumonia, and tuberculosis. Comfrey stimulates new cell growth and provides healing. It may be taken in capsules, if it is taken as a tea, use ¼ teaspoon of Comfrey herb powder to one cup of boiling water. Comfrey may be taken as often as you feel the need. For asthma it may be taken once or twice a day, for three to four days, or until desired results are reached. For some, two or three days a week can be helpful.

Contains: vitamins A, C, iron, sulphur, copper, zinc, magnesium, and Comfrey is very high in calcium, potassium, and protein.

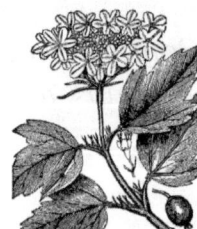

Cramp Bark

CRAMP BARK is a must-have for asthma. It is a sedative for the lungs and the nervous system. It treats abdominal cramps, uterine cramps, heart palpitations and hypertension. Cramp Bark may be taken in capsules. If it is taken as a tea, use ¼ teaspoon of Cramp Bark herb powder to one cup of boiling water. Cramp Bark may be taken as often as you feel the need. For asthma it may be taken once or twice a day, for three to five days, or until desired results are reached. For some, once or twice a week can be beneficial until desired results are reached.

Contains: calcium, potassium, magnesium, and Cramp Bark is very high in vitamins C and K.

| ASTHMA |

Damiana

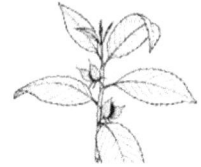

DAMIANA will assist treating asthma. It helps to overcome exhaustion and treats emphysema, depression, impotency, and infertility. It treats inflammation of the prostate, and Parkinson's disease and pulmonary disorders. Damiana is also an aphrodisiac and will enhance sexual desires in both men and women. It may be taken in capsules. If it is taken as a tea, use ¼ teaspoon of Damiana herb powder to one cup of boiling water. Damiana may be taken as often as you feel the need. For asthma it may be taken once or twice a day, for two to five days, or until desired results are reached. For some it may be taken once or twice a week for desired results.

Contains: vitamins A, C, and B complex, zinc, calcium, potassium, protein, selenium, and sodium.

**Dandelion*

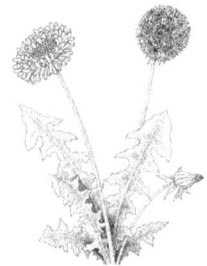

DANDELION can be a very good herb for treating asthma. It treats many aliments of the body and offers help fighting acne, anemia, and arthritis. It cleans the blood and promotes endurance. Dandelion treats kidney and liver problems. It is a diuretic and increases the flow of urine. It is high in organic sodium, and is helpful for treating calcium deficiencies. **Dandelion may elevate blood pressure for some people when taken excessively.** It is a bitter herb and it may be taken in capsules. If it is taken as a tea, use ¼ teaspoon of Dandelion herb powder to one cup of boiling water. Dandelion may be taken as often as you feel the need. For asthma it may be taken once or twice a day, for two to five days, or until desired results are reached. For some, once or twice a week can be beneficial until you are satisfied with the results.

Herbs for your blood type: Dandelion is highly beneficial for people with blood type O. It is neutral for people with blood type A, B, and AB.

Contains: calcium, vitamins A, B, C, and E, sodium, potassium, iron, nickel, tin, copper, magnesium, manganese, sulphur, and zinc.

ASTHMA

HERBS:

Elder Flower

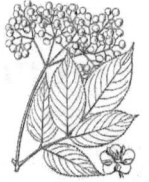

ELDER FLOWER acts as a sedative to relieve asthma. It clears the lungs, and when combined with Mullein, it helps to heal congestion. It will increase perspiration. Elder Flower is helpful when taken in the first stages of a cold. It treats pneumonia, allergies, bronchitis, colds, and sinus congestion. Elder Flower may be taken in capsules. If it is taken as a tea, use ¼ teaspoon of Elder Flower herb powder to one cup of boiling water. Elder Flower may be taken as often as you feel the need, for asthma it may be taken once or twice a day until desired results are reached. For some, once or twice a week can be helpful with prevention from time to time.

Herbs for your blood type: Elder Flower is neutral with people of blood type O, A, B and AB.

Contains: vitamins A and C.

Elecampane

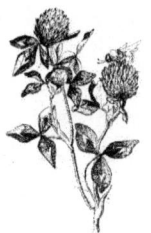

ELECAMPANE helps to treat asthma. It clears the lungs and respiratory organs. It removes phlegm, mucus and inflammation in the respiratory, it treats wheezing, coughs, and emphysema. It treats increase the appetite it treats bronchial ailments, and will lower sugar levels in the blood. It may be taken in capsules; if it is taken as a tea use ¼ teaspoon of Elecampane herb powder to one cup of boiling water. Elecampane may be taken as often as you feel the need. For asthma it may be taken once or twice a day until desired results are reached. For some, once or twice a week can be beneficial until results are reached.

Contains: sodium, calcium, and potassium.

ASTHMA

Eucalyptus

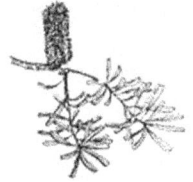

EUCALYPTUS will be helpful with treating asthma. Use it as a vapor. It treats respiratory infections, pneumonia, and congestion in the lungs.

Eucalyptus oil can be used as a steam inhalant, or it may be rubbed on the chest and back for relief for the lungs this book suggest that Eucalyptus is best used externally.

Fennel

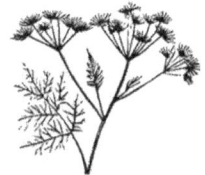

FENNEL will help with treating asthma. It will clear phlegm and mucus from the lungs, and helps to remove mucus in the intestinal tract. It is helpful for cancer patients after radiation and chemotherapy. For children it acts as a sedative, so you must use a smaller amount. It works well with other herbs and will curb the appetite. Urination will increase while using Fennel. It is a good herb to use as a spice in the kitchen. Fennel may be taken in capsules. If it is taken as a tea, use ¼ teaspoon of Fennel herb powder to one cup of boiling water. Fennel may be taken as often as you feel the need. For asthma it may be taken once or twice a day until desired results are reached. For some, once or twice a week can be helpful with prevention from time to time. Fennel may elevate blood pressure for some people when taken excessively.

Contains: sodium, potassium, sulphur, and is high in vitamin A.

Fenugreek

FENUGREEK will help to give relief from asthma. It treats mucus in the lungs, sinus problems, emphysema, infection and diabetes and dissolves cholesterol. Women who wish to get pregnant should not use fenugreek; it will impede the progress. Fenugreek is a pleasant tasting herb, and it may be taken in capsules. If it is taken as a tea, use ¼ teaspoon of Fenugreek herb powder to one cup of boiling water.

ASTHMA

HERBS:

Fenugreek may be taken as often as you feel the need. For asthma it may be taken once or twice a day, for three to four days, or until desired results are reached. For some once or twice a week can be helpful.

Herbs for your blood type: Fenugreek is highly beneficial for people with blood type O, and A. People with blood type B, or AB should avoid this herb.

Contains: vitamins B1, B2, iron, and choline. Fenugreek is very high in vitamins A and D.

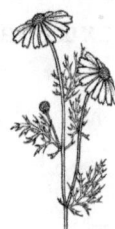

Feverfew

FEVERFEW will help to relieve asthma. It helps to treat the discomfort in the lungs. It treats colds, chills, and hay fever and gives relief from migraine headaches, sinus problems, and arthritis pain. **People with high blood pressure should not use this herb more than once a week: it may elevate blood pressure when taken excessively** It may be taken in capsules. If it is taken as a tea, use ¼ teaspoon of Feverfew herb powder to one cup of boiling water. Feverfew may be taken as often as you feel the need. For asthma it may be taken once or twice a day, for two to five days, or until desired results are reached. For some, once or twice a week can be helpful from time to time.

Contains: vitamins A and C, iron, niacin, potassium, selenium, sodium, and zinc.

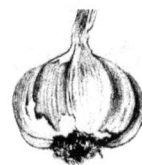

*Garlic

GARLIC can be great for treating asthma. It treats lung infections; it strengthens the immune system, and treats respiratory congestion. It treats coughs, colds, cancer, and fever. It reduces cholesterol. **Garlic may elevate blood pressure for some people when taken excessively.** It may be taken in capsules. If it is taken as a tea, use ¼ teaspoon of Garlic herb powder to one cup of boiling water. Garlic may be taken as often as you feel the need. For asthma it may be taken once or twice a day, for two to five days, or until desired results are reached. For some, once or twice a week can be beneficial for desired results.

ASTHMA

Herbs for your blood type: Garlic is highly beneficial for people with blood type A and AB. It is neutral for people with blood type O and B.

Contains: sodium, sulphur, calcium, copper, vitamin B1, iron, and is high in potassium, zinc, selenium, and vitamins A and C.

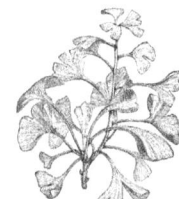

Ginkgo

GINKGO will reduce the frequency of attacks of asthma. It stimulates circulation, increases mental alertness, and the flow of oxygen to the brain. It improves hearing and it strengthens the retina in the eyes. It may be taken in capsules. If it is taken as a tea, use ¼ teaspoon of Ginkgo herb powder to one cup of boiling water. Ginkgo may be taken as often as you feel the need. For asthma it may be taken once or twice a day, for two to four days, or until desired results are reached. For some, once or twice a week can be helpful from time to time.

Contains bioflavonoids.

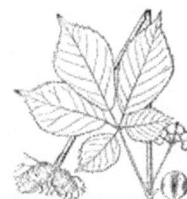

*Ginseng/Panax

GINSENG/PANAX can be an excellent herb for treating asthma. It strengthens the lungs, and combats chronic fatigue. It treats anemia, diabetes, chronic fever, and it stimulates the appetite. Some herbalist will use Ginseng/Panax to regulate blood pressure. Long-term use is not recommended for women, as it will produce testosterone. One week on and three weeks off will do fine for women. This herb will benefit men on long term just great! Ginseng/Panax is better prepared in glass cookware; metal pots will reduce the effects of the herbs. It may be taken in capsules, if it taken as a tea, use ¼ teaspoon of Ginseng/Panax herb powder to one cup of boiling water. Ginseng/Panax may be taken as often as you feel the need. For asthma it may be taken once a day, for two or four days, or until desired results are reached. For some, once or twice a week can be helpful from time to time.

Herbs for your blood type: Ginseng is highly beneficial for people with Blood types O, A, B, and AB.

Contains: vitamins A, E, and B 12, iron, sodium, calcium, potassium, sulphur, phosphorus, magnesium, and silicon.

ASTHMA

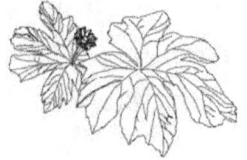

Golden Seal

GOLDEN SEAL will assist with the relief of asthma. It treats inflammation in the lungs, and strengthens the immune system. It clears the mucus membranes, treats colds, coughs, eye and ear infections. Golden Seal treats typhoid fever and wounds. It is a bitter tasting herb and will reduce sugar in the blood when it is used with the Licorice herb. Use Myrrh if there is low blood sugar. Do not take this herb if you are pregnant. Golden Seal may be taken in capsules, if it taken as a tea, use ¼ teaspoon of Golden Seal herb powder to one cup of boiling water. Golden Seal may be taken as often as you feel the need. For asthma it may be taken once or twice a day, for two to five days, or until desired results are reached. For some, once or twice a week can be beneficial. People with high blood pressure should not use this herb more than once a week.

   Herbs for your blood type: Golden Seal is neutral for people of blood type A, B and AB. This herb should be avoided for people with blood type O.

Contains: calcium, potassium, iron, zinc, sodium, and vitamins A, C, B complex, and E.

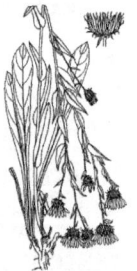

*Gumweed

GUMWEED offers great benefits for asthma. It treats the lungs and will treat the wheezing caused by asthma. For internal use, Use a very small amount mixed with another asthma fighting herb. **Gumweed is not recommended for people with heart problems.** Use less than 1/8th teaspoon of this herb to one cup of boiling water. Gumweed may be taken once a day for not more than two days a week, until desired results are reached.

Contains: lead, tin, zinc, and some arsenic.

ASTHMA

HERBS:

*Horehound

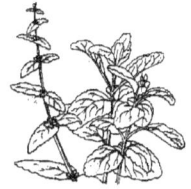

HOREHOUND will remove phlegm from the respiratory system. It is highly recommended for lung relief. It treats colds, coughs, and hepatitis. Large amounts of Horehound at one time will act as a laxative.

It may be taken in capsules. If it is taken as a tea, use ¼ teaspoon of Horehound herb powder to one cup of boiling water. Horehound may be taken as often as you feel the need. For chronic asthma it may be taken once or twice a day, for two to five days, or until desired results are reached. For some, once or twice a week can be beneficial.

Herbs for your blood type: Horehound is neutral for people with blood type O, A, B and AB.

Contains: iron, potassium, sulphur, and vitamins A, E, C, and B complex.

*Horseradish

HORSERADISH can be great for treating sufferers of asthma. It does wonders for upper respiratory problems, and it relieves water retention. Horseradish stimulates the appetite. It may be taken in capsules. If this herb is taken as a tea, use ¼ teaspoon of Horseradish herb powder to one cup of boiling water. Horseradish may be taken as often as you feel the need. For chronic asthma it may be taken once or twice a day, for two to five days, or until desired results are reached. For some, once or twice a week can be beneficial from time to time.

Contains: vitamins A, B complex, iron, calcium, sodium, and phosphorus.

Hyssop

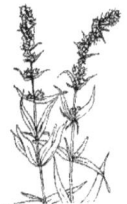

HYSSOP can be helpful for treating asthma. It removes mucus and phlegm from the lungs, strengthens the immune system, and it will do wonders to stop the wheezing

---
ASTHMA
---

of asthma. Hyssop may be taken in capsules. If it is taken as a tea, use ¼ teaspoon of Hyssop herb powder to one cup of boiling water. Hyssop may be taken as often as you feel the need. For asthma it may be taken once or twice a day, for three to four days, or until desired results are reached. For some, once or twice a week can be helpful from time to time.

Contains: nutrients of sulfur, flavonoids, marrubin, and tannins.

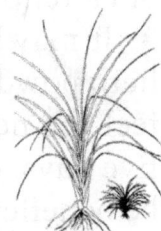

Lemon Grass

LEMON GRASS will help to treat asthma. It will reduce mucus in the respiratory system. For infants and children use a smaller amount. It helps when there is a cold. It will increase urination and help to treat internal parasites. Lemon Grass may be taken in capsules. If it is taken as a tea, use ¼ teaspoon of Lemon Grass herb powder to one cup of boiling water. Lemon Grass may be taken as often as you feel the need. For asthma it may be taken once or twice a day, for two to four days, or until desired results are reached. For some, once or twice a week can be beneficial.

Contains: calcium, iron, magnesium, manganese, phosphorus, potassium, selenium, and zinc, and is high in vitamins A and C

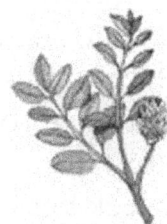

Licorice

LICORICE will assist with treating asthma. It expels phlegm from the lungs, helps with allergies, treats Addison disease, and arthritis. It increases energy; treats weight loss, and gastrointestinal problems. Licorice works as a laxative; and contains a natural hormone that replaces cortisone in the body. It is a bitter herb and it may be taken in capsules. If it is taken as a tea, use ¼ teaspoon Licorice herb powder to one cup of boiling water. Licorice may be taken as often as you feel the need. For asthma it may be taken once or twice a day, for two to five days, or until desired results are reached. For some, once or twice a week from time to time can be beneficial.

ASTHMA

HERBS:

Herbs for your Blood type: Licorice is highly beneficial for people with blood type B and AB. It is compatible for people with blood type O and A.
Contains: niacin, lecithin, iodine, chromium, zinc, and vitamins E and B complex.

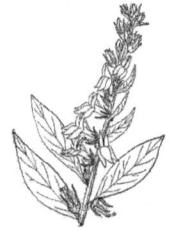

*Lobelia

LOBELIA can be very beneficial for treating chronic asthma. It treats lung problems, relaxes the nervous system and increases urine flow. It treats allergies, bursitis, and St. Vitus' Dance (Chorea). It is a bitter herb and it may be taken in capsules, if it is taken as a tea, use ¼ teaspoon of Lobelia herb powder to one cup of boiling water. Lobelia may be taken as often as you feel the need. For chronic asthma problems it may be taken once or twice a day, for two to five days, or until desired results are reached. For some, two or three times a week can be beneficial from time to time.

Contains: iron, copper, sodium, sulphur, cobalt, lead, and selenium.
LOTS OF WATER SHOULD BE TAKEN WITH LOBELIA.

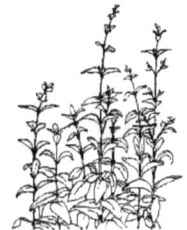

Marjoram

MARJORAM will be helpful for treating asthma. It treats respiratory problems; violent convulsions, abdominal cramps, colic, measles, whooping cough and vomiting. Marjoram can be kept in the kitchen as a spice for cooking. Marjoram should not be used while pregnant. It may be taken in capsules, if it is taken as a tea, use ¼ teaspoon of Marjoram herb powder to one cup of boiling water. Marjoram may be taken as often as you feel the need. For asthma it may be taken once or twice a day, for two to three days, or until desired results are reached. For some, once or twice a week can be helpful from time to time.

Herbs for your Blood type: Marjoram is neutral for people with blood type O, A, B and AB.

Contains: sodium, iron, potassium, magnesium, zinc, calcium, niacin, silicon, and vitamins A and C.

ASTHMA

HERBS:

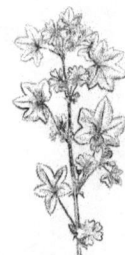

*Marshmallow

MARSHMALLOW works exceptionally well for treating asthma. It treats emphysema and the upper respiratory system. It removes mucus from the lungs. Marshmallow may elevate blood pressure for some people when taken excessively. It is a pleasant tasting herb and it may be taken in capsules, if it is taken as a tea, use ¼ teaspoon of Marshmallow herb powder to one cup of boiling water. Marshmallow may be taken as often as you feel the need. For asthma it may be taken once a day for three to seven days, or until desired results are reached. For some it may be taken once or twice a week can be beneficial from time to time.

Do not confuse Marshmallow herb with the candy like marshmallow found in the food section of the market.

Contains: sodium, iodine, B complex, and pantothenic acid. It is high in vitamin A and calcium, zinc, and iron.

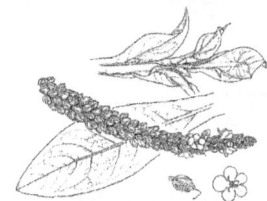

Mullein

MULLEIN will assist with treating asthma. It loosens and removes excess mucus from the system. It treats bleeding lungs, allergies and respiratory problems. It treats emphysema and sinus problems. Mullein also has a calming effect on the nervous system. **Mullein is best taken at bedtime because it will cause sleepiness.** It may be taken in capsules. If Mullein it is taken as a tea. Use ¼ teaspoon of Mullein herb powder to one cup of boiling water. Mullein may be taken as often as you feel the need. For asthma it may be taken once or twice a day, for two to five days, or until desired results are reached. For some, once or twice a week can be helpful.

Herbs for your blood type: Mullein is neutral for people with blood type O and A. People with Blood type B and AB should avoid this herb.

Contains: magnesium, potassium, and sulphur, and is very high in iron.

ASTHMA

*Myrrh

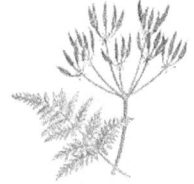

MYRRH can be an excellent choice for treating chronic asthma. It is very effective in removing mucus and treating lung diseases. Myrrh will also stimulate and promote menstruation. Myrrh has antiseptic properties and it may be used in place of Golden Seal. Myrrh is a bitter herb and it may be taken in capsules. If it is taken as a tea, use, ¼ teaspoon of Myrrh herb powder to one cup of boiling water. Myrrh may be taken as often as you feel the need. For chronic asthma it may be taken once or twice a day, for two to five days, or until desired results are reached. For some, once or twice a week can be beneficial.

Contains: potassium, sodium, chlorine, silicon, and zinc.

Nettle

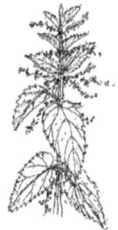

NETTLE will assist with the relief of asthma. It treats respiratory infections, internal bleeding, hives, and urinary infections. Nettle will increase thyroid functioning. Nettle treats scalp infections, and baldness. Nettle is a pleasant tasting herb. It may be taken in capsules. If it is taken as a tea, use ¼ teaspoon of Nettle herb powder to one cup of boiling water. Nettle may be taken as often as you feel the need. For asthma it may be taken once a day for two to five days, or until desired results are reached. For some, once or twice a week can be helpful.

Contains: vitamins A, C, D, E, F, and P, copper, potassium, sodium, calcium, chlorophyll, sulphur, silicon, protein, and zinc, and is high in iron and minerals.

ASTHMA

Parsley

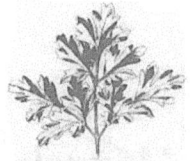

PARSLEY will assist with treating respiratory problems. It treats allergies, halitosis and it is a diuretic. It will be helpful when urination is painful. Parsley when used in large amounts for a long period, will sweeten the breath. Do not use Parsley during pregnancy it will induce labor pains. However, after birth it will dry up mother's milk during the weaning period. It may be taken in capsules. If it is taken as a tea, use ¼ teaspoons of Parsley herb powder to one cup of boiling water. Parsley may be taken as often as you feel the need. For treating asthma it may be taken once a day for two to five days, or until desired results are reached. For some, Use once or twice a week can be helpful.

Herbs for your blood type: Parsley is highly beneficial for blood type O and B. It is neutral with blood type A and AB.

Contains: vitamins A, B, and C, chlorophyll, iron, potassium, calcium, cobalt, copper, riboflavin, silicon, sodium, sulphur, and thiamine.

Pau D'Arco

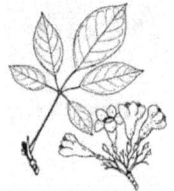

PAU D'ARCO can be helpful with treating asthma; it treats respiratory problems, AIDS, allergies, esophagus, parasites and tumors. Pau D'Arco has many benefits. It has great cancer fighting abilities as well. It may be taken in capsules. If it is taken as a tea, use ¼ teaspoon of Pau D'Arco herb powder to one cup of boiling water. Pau D'Arco may be taken as often as you feel the need. For treating asthma it may be taken once a day for two to four days, or until desired results are reached. For some, once a week can be beneficial.

Contains: potassium, sodium, magnesium, manganese, selenium, and zinc. Vitamins A, B complex, and C. Pau D'Arco is very high in iron.

ASTHMA

*Pleurisy Root

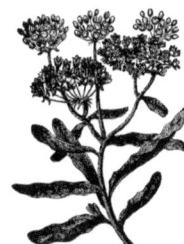

PLEURISY ROOT is excellent for treating asthma. It treats breathing problems, clears the lungs and improves oxygen intake. It helps to clear thick mucus, inflammation and phlegm. Vitamin C should be taken when using this herb. Do not use Pleurisy Root if you suffer a weak pulse and cold skin; Yarrow may be used instead. Pleurisy Root relaxes the whole body. **Pleurisy Root is not recommended for children. Using large amounts of Pleurisy may be toxic to the body. Do not use Pleurisy during pregnancy: it may induce spontaneous abortion. Do not use while breast-feeding. Do not use Pleurisy if there is a history of heart disease or certain types of cancer.** It may be taken in capsules, if it is taken as a tea, use 1/8th teaspoon or less of Pleurisy Root herb powder to one cup of boiling water. Pleurisy Root may be taken as often as you feel the need. For treating asthma it may be taken once a day for two to three days, or until desired results are reached. For some, once or twice a week can be.

Prickly Ash

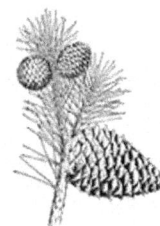

PRICKLY ASH will help with the relief of asthma. It treats a wide variety of conditions. It treats fevers, mouth sores, syphilis, and stimulates and increases the flow of saliva in the mouth. Prickly Ash will increase circulation to the legs. It warms cold hands, cold feet, and cold legs. It may cause some people to become more sensitive to sunlight and burn more easily. It helps to treat yeast growth and gonorrhea. Prickly Ash may be taken in capsules. If it is taken as a tea, use ¼ teaspoon of Prickly ash herb powder to one cup of boiling water. Prickly may be taken as often as you feel the need. For asthma it may be taken once or twice a day, for two to four days, or until desired results are reached. For some, two or three times a week can be helpful.

Contains tannins.

ASTHMA

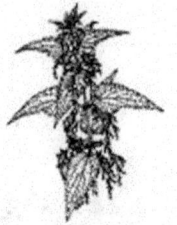

Saw Palmetto

SAW PALMETTO helps to give relief from asthma. It treats lung congestion and whooping cough. Saw Palmetto is a sexual stimulant. It treats frigidity and impotency and the bladder. It reduces enlarged prostate glands. It may be taken in capsules. If it is taken as a tea, use ¼ teaspoon of Saw Palmetto herb powder to one cup of boiling water. Saw Palmetto may be taken as often as you feel the need. For asthma it may be taken once a day for two to three days, or until desired results are reached. For some, once or twice a week can be helpful for desired results.

Contains vitamin A.

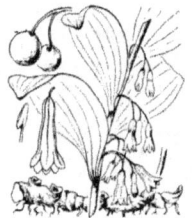

Schizandra

SCHIZANDRA can be helpful for treating asthma. It treats lung problems, strengthens the immune system and helps with nervous conditions. Schizandra increases contractions of the heart muscle, and enhances sexual desires. Schizandra is a tonic that increases energy, treats fatigue, and impotency. It may be taken in capsules. If it is taken as a tea, use ¼ teaspoon of Schizandra herb powder to one cup of boiling water. Schizandra may be taken as often as you feel the need. For asthma it may be taken once or twice a day for two to five days, or until desired results are reached,

Contains: magnesium, calcium, iron, vitamin C, potassium, and sodium.

ASTHMA

Seneca

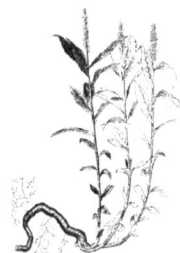

SENECA will help to give relief for asthma. It removes phlegm from the lungs; it eases respiratory problems, treats pneumonia and small pox. Seneca may be taken in capsules, if it is taken as a tea, add ¼ teaspoon of Seneca powder herb to one cup of boiling water. Seneca may be taken as often as you feel the need. For asthma it may be taken once or twice a day, for two to five days, or until desired results are reached. For some, once or twice a week can be helpful.

Contains: iron, lead, tin, aluminum, and magnesium.

*Slippery Elm

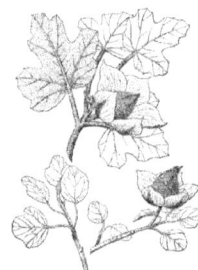

SLIPPERY ELM can be great for treating asthma. It is of great benefit to the lungs. It will smooth bowel eliminations as well. Slippery Elm should be taken in capsules because it will not dissolve in liquid. Slippery Elm may be taken as often as you feel the need. For asthma it may be taken once a day for two to four days, or until desired results are reached. For some, once a week can be helpful.

Herbs for your blood type: Slippery Elm is highly beneficial for people with blood type O, and blood type A. It is neutral for people with blood type B and AB.

Contains: iron, sodium, iodine, zinc, copper, potassium, vitamins K and E.

ASTHMA

HERBS:

Thyme

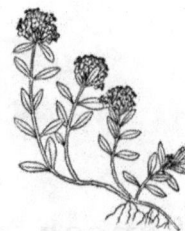

THYME will help with treating asthma. It is very good for the lungs when there is shortness of the breath. It has also been known to kill worms in the stomach. Thyme can be kept in the kitchen and used as a spice. **Thyme may elevate blood pressure for some people when taken excessively.** If there is hypertension it should not be used more than once a week. It may be taken in capsules. It is taken as a tea, use ¼ teaspoon of Thyme herb powder to one cup of boiling water. Thyme may be taken as often as you feel the need. For treating asthma it may be taken once a day for two to four days, or until desired results are reached. For some, once a week can be beneficial.

Herbs for your blood type: Thyme is highly beneficial for people with blood type O and B. It is neutral for people with blood type A and AB.

Contains: sodium, iodine, sulphur, and vitamins C and D.

*Violet

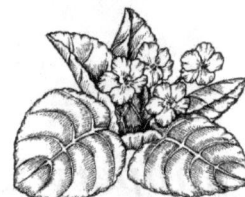

VIOLET is an excellent herb for treating asthma. It is an herb that asthma patients should never be without. It treats respiratory disorders and chronic asthma coughs. Phlegm quickly disappears from the lungs. It will eliminate the difficulty of breathing. Violet is a pleasant tasting herb. It may be taken in capsules, if it is taken as a tea, use ¼ teaspoon of Violet herb powder to one cup of boiling water. Violet may be taken as often as you feel the need. For asthma it may be taken once or twice a day, for two to seven days, or until desired results are reached. For some, once or twice a week will be beneficial.

Contains: vitamins A and C.

ASTHMA

HERBS:

*Wild Cherry

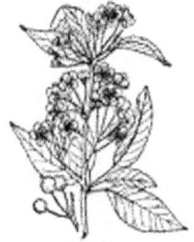

WILD CHERRY is a must-have for treating asthma. It removes mucus and phlegm very well. It calms the nerves and coughs. It is a remedy for heart palpitations. It will increase the appetite. It may be taken in capsules. If it is taken as a tea, use ¼ teaspoon of Wild Cherry herb powder to one cup of boiling water. Wild Cherry may be taken as often as you feel the need. For treating asthma it may be taken once or twice a day, for two to five days, or until desired results are reached. For some, once or twice a week can be helpful.

Contains: calcium, iron, magnesium, phosphorus, potassium, and zinc.

*WildYam

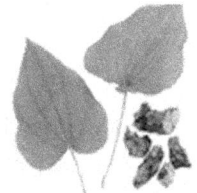

WILD YAM is among the best herbs for treating asthma. It treats lung congestion, calms the nervous system and stops the cough that causes discomfort to asthma sufferers. It treats Addison's disease, increases energy, assists with weight loss, and gastrointestinal problems. Wild Yam may be taken in capsules, if it is taken as a tea, use ¼ teaspoon of Wild Yam herb powder to one cup of boiling water. Wild may be taken as often as you feel the need. For asthma it may be taken once or twice a day, for two to four days, or until desired results are reached. For some once or twice a week will be beneficial.

Contains: vitamins A, B complex, and C, iron, potassium, sodium, phosphorus, calcium, silicon, magnesium, and manganese.

ASTHMA

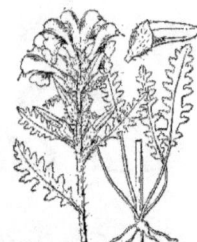

Wood Betony

WOOD BETONY will aid with bronchial asthma. It is excellent for treating nervous conditions, epilepsy and Parkinson's disease. Wood Betony is soothing for children as well as adults. Wood Betony will increase urination. It is a bitter herb and it may be taken in capsules. If it is taken as a tea; use ¼ teaspoon of Wood Betony herb powder to one cup of boiling water. Wood Betony may be taken as often as you feel the need. For asthma it may be taken once or twice a day, for two to five days, or until desired results are reached. For some, once or twice a week can be helpful.

Contains vitamin C, manganese, and phosphorus.

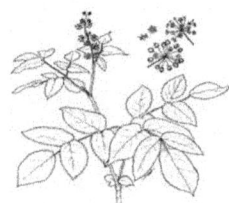

*Yerba Santa

YERBA SANTA is excellent for treating chronic or acute asthma. It stimulates the lungs and expels mucus. It treats allergies, bronchial congestion, and hay fever. This is a bitter herb. It may be taken in capsules. If it is taken as a tea, use ¼ teaspoon of Yerba Santa herb powder to one cup of boiling water. Yerba Santa may be taken as often as you feel the need. For asthma it may be taken once or twice days for two to five days, or until desired results are reached. For some, once or twice a week can be useful.

Contains: potassium, selenium, sodium, zinc, and vitamin A.

BLADDER

Agrimony

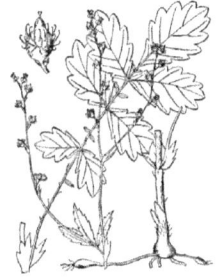

AGRIMONY helps to remove stones or gravel from the bladder. It will treat the kidneys, incontinence, urination and uterine bleeding. Agrimony is high in nutrients and it is a tonic. It is a pleasant tasting herb and may be taken in capsules. If it is taken as a tea, use ¼ teaspoon of Agrimony herb powder to one cup of boiling water. Agrimony may be taken as often as you feel the need. For bladder problems it may be taken once or twice a day for three to five days, or day until desired results are reached. For some, two or three times a week can be beneficial.

Contains: iron, niacin, vitamin K, and B3.

Alfalfa

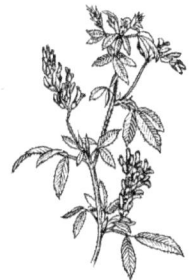

ALFALFA will be helpful for treating the bladder. It will remove inflammation in the bladder, it cleans the kidneys and the liver. It treats jaundice and acidity. Alfalfa can be helpful for the prevention of colon cancer when taken over an extended period. Alfalfa is a pleasant tasting herb and it may be taken in capsules. If it is taken as a tea, use ¼ teaspoon of Alfalfa herb powder to one cup of boiling water. Alfalfa may be taken as often as you feel the need. For treating the bladder it may be taken two or three times a day, for two to five days, or until desired results are reached. For some, two or three times a week can be beneficial.

Herbs for your blood type: Alfalfa is highly beneficial for people with blood type A. And it is neutral for people with blood type B and AB. People with blood type O should avoid this herb it will cause excessive blood thinning for them.

BLADDER

Contains: vitamins A, B complex, D, E, and K, iron, potassium, magnesium, protein, sodium, sulfur, and phosphorus. Alfalfa is very high in calcium, chlorophyll, and vitamin B12.

Astragalus

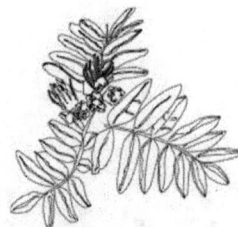

ASTRAGALUS will reduce infections of the bladder. It treats the kidneys, improves urine flow, and increases energy. It helps to eliminate toxins in the body and promotes healing of damaged tissues. It strengthens T-cells and helps to lower blood pressure. Urination will increase while using Astragalus. Astragalus may be taken in capsules. If it is taken as a tea, use ¼ teaspoons of Astragalus herb powder to one cup of boiling water. Astragalus may be taken as often as you feel the need. For treating the bladder it may be taken once or twice a day for four to five days or until desired results are reached. For some, once or twice a week can be beneficial.

Contains: choline, betaine, and gluconic acid.

Barberry

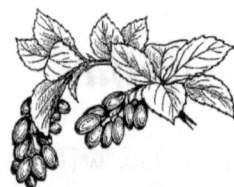

BARBERRY will help to treat the bladder. It treats the kidneys, liver and a sluggish gallbladder. Barberry works best when used with other herbs. Do not take Barberry excessively; it may cause depression. It dilates blood vessels, which makes it a good choice for treating high blood pressure. Barberry is a bitter herb and it may be taken in capsules, if it is taken as a tea, use 1/8th teaspoon or less of Barberry herb powder to one cup of boiling water. Barberry may be taken as often as you feel the need. For bladder problems it may be taken once or twice a day for two to five days or until desired results are reached. For some, once or twice a week will help to give relief.

Contains: iron, manganese, phosphorus, and vitamin C.

BLADDER

Basil

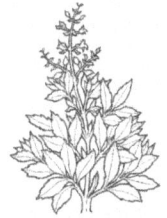

BASIL can be helpful for treating the bladder. It treats kidney and liver problems. It treats headaches, indigestion and parasites. Basil is best-used fresh in salads and other food preparations. It will stimulate and promote energy. Basil can be taken in capsules. If it is taken as a tea, use ¼ teaspoon of Basil herb powder to one cup of boiling water. Basil may be taken as often as you feel the need. For bladder problems it may be taken once or twice a day, for two to seven days, or until desired results are reached. For some, once or twice a week will be helpful.

Herbs for your Blood type: Basil is neutral for people with blood type O, A, B, and AB.

Contains: iron, calcium, magnesium, phosphorus, and vitamins A, D, and B2.

*Bilberry

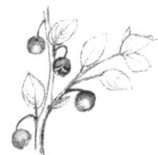

BILBERRY can be an excellent herb for treating the bladder. It removes stones in the bladder, and treats kidney problems. It will help to treat urinary problems, and infections. It will be helpful during pregnancy to strengthen the veins. Bilberry is best used in combination with other herbs.

Bilberry may be taken in capsules, if it is taken as a tea use 1/8th teaspoon, or less, of Bilberry herb powder to one cup of boiling water. Bilberry may be taken as often as you feel the need. For treating the bladder it may be taken once or twice a day for two to five days or until desired results are reached. For some, once or twice a week can be beneficial.

Contains: manganese, iron, zinc, potassium, calcium, sodium, and selenium.

BLADDER

*Birch

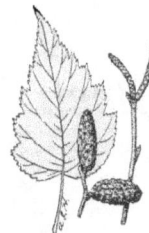

BIRCH can be very effective in relieving pain in the bladder. It is one of the things Birch does best. It treats arthritis, and rheumatism. Birch is a sedative and should be taken at bedtime. It may be taken in capsules, if it is taken as a tea use ¼ teaspoon of Birch herb powder to one cup of boiling water. Birch may be taken as often as you feel the need. For bladder pain it may be taken once or twice a day, for three to seven days or until desired results are reached. For some, once or twice a week will be beneficial.

Contains: calcium, sodium, potassium, iron, magnesium, copper, chlorine, and vitamins A, B1, B2, C, and E.

Black Walnut

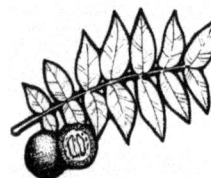

BLACK WALNUT can be useful for treating the bladder. It treats urinary problems. Black Walnut offers treatments for cancer, lupus, and vaginal discharge. It has a high organic iodine content. Black Walnut may be taken in capsules. If it is taken as a tea, use ¼ teaspoon of Black Walnut herb powder to one cup of boiling water. Black Walnut may be taken as often as you feel the need. For treating the bladder and urinary problems it may be taken once or twice a day for three to five days or until desired results are reached. For some once or twice a week can be helpful.

Contains: vitamins A, B1, B2, B6, C, P, magnesium, potassium, iron, calcium manganese, niacin, organic iodine, phosphorus, potassium, selenium, bioflavonoids, and B15.

BLADDER

*Blue Vervain

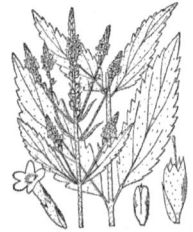

BLUE VERVAIN offers recovery for the bladder. It treats uterine problems and has a soothing and calming tranquilizing effect to the entire body. It treats poor circulation, fevers, insomnia and a toxic liver. Large amounts of this herb taken at once may cause vomiting. It is a pleasant tasting herb and it may be taken in capsules. If it is taken as a tea, use ¼ teaspoon of Blue Vervain herb powder to one cup of boiling water. Blue Vervain may be taken as often as you feel the need. For treating the bladder it may be taken once or twice a day for two to six days, or until desired relief are reached. For some, once or twice a week can offer relief.

Contains: vitamin C, calcium, manganese, and vitamin E.

Borage

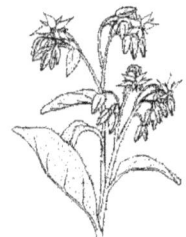

BORAGE will assist with the bladder. It treats kidney problems; it strengthens the heart and acts as a tonic for the entire body. Borage may be taken in capsules. If it is taken as a tea, use ¼ teaspoon of Borage herb powder to one cup of boiling water. Borage may be taken as often as you feel the need. For treating the bladder it may be taken once or twice a day for two to five days or until desired results are reached. For some, once or twice a week can assist with treatment.

Contains: calcium and potassium.

BLADDER

*Buchu Leaf

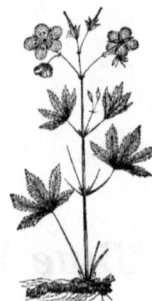

BUCHU LEAF treats inflammation in the bladder. It treats kidney problems, prostate problems, venereal disease, and urinary tract infections. It reduces pain when urinating. Urination increases without the pain. Buchu Leaf can be taken in capsules. If it is taken as a tea, use ¼ teaspoon of Buchu herb powder to one cup of boiling water. Buchu Leaf may be taken as often as you feel the need. For bladder irritation it may be taken once or twice a day for two to five days or until desired results are reached. For some, once or twice a week will offer results.

Burdock

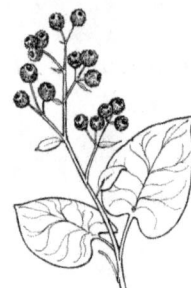

BURDOCK will treat infection in the bladder. It helps to promote kidney functioning, and it treats cancer, bursitis, and constipation. It treats swelling and fluid retention. Burdock contains a high amount of insulin.

Do not use an excessive amount of Burdock at once, it may cause vomiting. It may be taken in capsules. If it is taken as a tea, use ¼ teaspoon of Burdock herb powder to one cup of boiling water. Burdock may be taken as often as you feel the need. For bladder infections it may be taken once or twice a day for two to five days or until desired results are reached. For some once or twice a week will be beneficial.

Herbs for your Blood type: Burdock is highly beneficial for people with blood type A and AB. It is neutral for people with blood type B. People with blood type O should avoid this herb it will cause excessive blood thinning and excessive bleeding.

Contains: vitamins A, B complex, C, and E, iron, zinc, and sulphur.

BLADDER

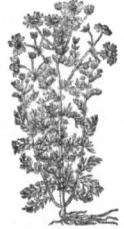

Chamomile

CHAMOMILE will assist with treating inflammation in the bladder. It treats the spleen, and peptic ulcers, bronchitis, poor circulation, fevers and drug addictions. It is a sedative and it is best taken at bedtime, it will relax the system. Chamomile will stimulate the appetite. Chamomile can be taken in capsules, if it is taken as a tea, use ¼ teaspoon of Chamomile herb powder to one cup of boiling water. Chamomile may be taken as often as you feel the need. For treating the bladder it may be taken once or twice a day for two to five days or until desired results are reached. For some, once or twice a week will assist.

Herbs for your Blood type: Chamomile is highly beneficial for people with blood type A and AB. It is neutral for people with blood type O and B.

Contains: potassium, calcium, iron, manganese, vitamin A, and zinc.

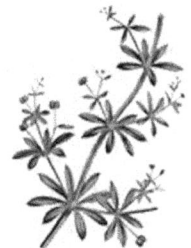

Cleavers

CLEAVERS will assist with treating stones and gravel in the bladder.

It may be taken in capsules, if it is taken as a tea, use ¼ teaspoon of Cleavers herb powder to one cup of boiling water. Cleavers may be taken as often as you feel the need. For stones or gravel in the bladder it may be taken once or twice a day for two to five days or until desired results are reached. For some, once or twice a week will assist with treatment.

BLADDER

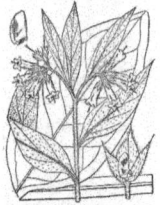

*Comfrey

COMFREY can be very beneficial for treating the bladder. It treats infections, blood in the urine, and pain. It treats cancer, emphysema pneumonia, and tuberculosis. Comfrey stimulates new cell growth and provides healing. Comfrey may be taken in capsules, if it is taken as a tea use ¼ teaspoon of Comfrey herb powder to one cup of boiling water. Comfrey may be taken as often as you feel the need. For treating the bladder it may be taken once or twice a day for one to five days or until desired results are reached. For some, two or three times a week can be helpful until desired results are reached.

Contains: vitamins A and C, iron, sulphur, copper, zinc, magnesium, and Comfrey is very high in calcium, potassium, and protein.

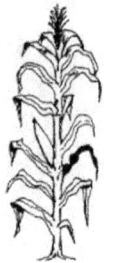

*Cornsilk

CORNSILK can be useful for treating an acutely inflamed bladder. It treats painful urination, kidney problems, prostate problems, cholesterol and gonorrhea. It is a diuretic. Cornsilk may be taken in capsules, if it is taken as a tea use 1/8th teaspoon or less of Cornsilk herb powder to one cup of boiling water. Cornsilk may be taken as often as you feel the need. For an inflamed bladder it may be taken once or twice a day for one to seven days or until desired results are reached. For some, once or twice a week will be beneficial.

Contains: vitamin B, silicon, and is very high in vitamin K.

BLADDER

Damiana

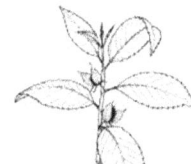

DAMIANA will help to treat inflammation in the bladder. It treats female problems, frigidity, and inflammation in the prostate. It balances hormones for men and women. Damiana is an aphrodisiac and will enhance sexual desires in both men and women. Damiana may be taken in capsules. If it is taken as a tea, use ¼ teaspoon of Damiana herb powder to one cup of boiling water. Damiana may be taken as often as you feel the need. For treating the bladder it may be taken once or twice a day for one to five days or until desired results are reached. For some, once or twice a week can be beneficial.

Contains: vitamins A, C, zinc, B complex, calcium, potassium, protein, selenium, and sodium.

Dandelion

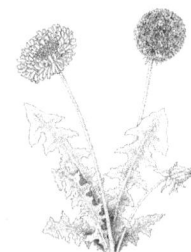

DANDELION will help to treat the bladder. It treats kidney infections, liver problems, and it lowers cholesterol, it treats breast cancer and stimulates the appetite. Dandelion will increase urine flow, and remove stiffness from the joints. **Dandelion may elevate blood pressure for some people when taken excessively.** Dandelion may be taken in capsules. If it is taken as a tea, use ¼ teaspoon of Dandelion herb powder to one cup of boiling water. Dandelion may be taken as often as you feel the need. For treating bladder problems it may be taken once or twice a day for two to five days or until desired results are reached. For some, once or twice a week can be helpful.

Herbs for your Blood type: Dandelion is highly beneficial for people with blood type O. It is neutral for people with blood type A, B, and AB.

Contains: calcium, vitamin A, B, C, E, sodium, potassium, iron, nickel, tin, copper magnesium, manganese, sulphur, and zinc.

BLADDER

HERBS:

*Devil's Claw

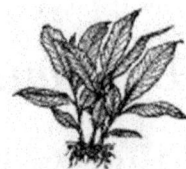

DEVIL'S CLAW strengthens the bladder. It strengthens the kidneys treats liver disease and back pain, it helps with aging problems. It treats cholesterol, and diabetes. It gives the body an all around overhaul. Devil's Claw may be taken in capsules. If it is taken as a tea, use ¼ teaspoon of Devil's Claw herb powder to one cup of boiling water. Devil's Claw may be taken as often as you feel the need. For treating the bladder it may be taken once or twice a day for two to five days or until desired results are reached. For some, two or three times a week can be beneficial.

Contains: Calcium, iron, magnesium, manganese, phosphorus, potassium, protein, selenium, silicon, sodium, vitamins A, C, and zinc.

Echinacea

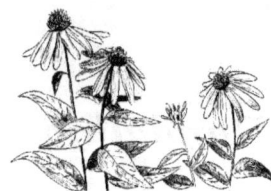

ECHINACEA will assist with treating infection in the bladder. It treats cancer; it cleans and purifies the blood. It treats the prostate glands and syphilis. Echinacea is an antibiotic and it increases white blood cells. Echinacea may be taken in capsules. If it is taken as tea, use ¼ teaspoon of Echinacea herb powder to one cup of boiling water. Echinacea may be taken as often as you feel the need. For bladder infections it may be taken once or twice a day for three to seven days or until desired results are reached. For some, two or three times a week can be beneficial.

   Herbs for your blood type: Echinacea is highly beneficial for people with blood type A and AB. It is neutral for people with blood type B. People with blood type O should avoid this herb. Echinacea will cause excessive blood thinning for people with blood type O.

Contains: vitamins A, C, E, iron, iodine, copper, sulphur, and potassium.

BLADDER

HERBS:

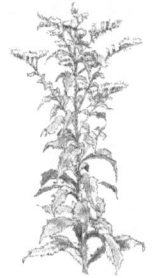

Golden Rod

GOLDEN ROD will help to remove stones in the bladder. It treats the kidneys, and urinary problems, it will clear up dark cloudy urine. Golden Rod may be taken in capsules. If it is taken as tea, use, ¼ teaspoon of Golden Rod herb powder to one cup of boiling water. Golden Rod may be taken as often as you feel the need. For stones in the bladder it may be taken once or twice a day for two to five days or until desired results are reached. For some, once or twice a week for a couple of weeks, or longer if you feel the need.

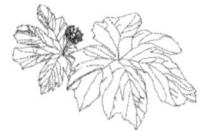

*Golden Seal

GOLDEN SEAL treats infections in the bladder. It treats internal bleeding, kidney and liver problems. Golden Seal treats prostate glands and venereal disease. Golden Seal will reduce sugar in the blood when it is used with the Licorice herb. Use Myrrh with Golden Seal if there is a low blood sugar. **Golden Seal may elevate blood pressure for some people. Do not take this herb if you are pregnant.** Golden Seal may be taken in capsules. If it is taken as a tea, use ¼ teaspoon of Golden Seal herb powder to one cup of boiling water. Golden Seal may be taken as often as you feel the need. For chronic bladder problems it may be taken once or twice a day for two to five days or until desired results are reached. For some, two or three times a week will be beneficial.

Herbs for your Blood type: Golden Seal is neutral for people with blood type A, B and AB. People with blood type O should avoid this herb it will over stimulate the immune system and cause a blood thinning problem for blood type O.

Contains: sodium, calcium, potassium, iron, zinc, and vitamins A, C, B complex, and E.

BLADDER

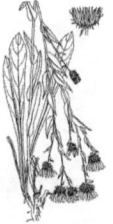

Gumweed

GUMWEED is excellent for treating infections in the bladder. It treats uterine infections, asthma and bronchitis. Gumweed should be used in combination with other herbs. **Gumweed is not recommended for people with heart problems.** It may be taken in capsules. If it is taken as a tea, use 1/8th teaspoon of Gumweed herb powder or less to one cup of boiling water. Gumweed may be taken as often as you feel the need. For treating the bladder it may be taken once a day for two to five days, or until desired results are reached. For some, once a week can be beneficial for two or three weeks can be beneficial.

Contains: lead, tin, zinc, and some arsenic.

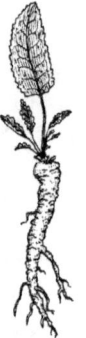

Horseradish

HORSERADISH is a good herb to use for the bladder. It treats urinary problems. Horseradish stimulates the appetite and treats poor circulation, digestive disorders and the liver. Use Horseradish in combination with other herbs for bladder problems. It may be taken in capsules. If it is taken as a tea, use ¼ teaspoon of Horseradish herb powder to one cup of boiling water. Horseradish may be taken as often as you feel the need. For treating the bladder it may be taken once or twice a day for two to five days or until desired results are reached. For some, once or twice a week can be helpful for prevention.

Contains: vitamins A, B complex, iron, calcium, sodium, and phosphorus.

BLADDER

Horsetail

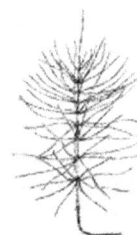

HORSETAIL can be a great for treating the bladder. It treats kidney problems and it eliminates urinary ulcers and gives a very easy urinary flow. It treats poor circulation and diabetes. Horsetail is excellent for hair and fingernail growth. **Horsetail may elevate blood pressure for some people when taken excessively.** People with high blood pressure should not take horsetail more than once a week. If it must be taken, use only a pinch in combination with other herbs. It may be taken in capsules. If it is taken as a tea, use ¼ teaspoon of Horsetail herb powder to one cup of boiling water. Horsetail may be taken as often as you feel the need. For treating the bladder it may be taken once or twice a day for two to five days or until desired results are reached. For some, two or three times a week can be beneficial.

Contains: sodium, iron, iodine, copper, vitamin E, and a high amount of silicon and selenium.

Hydrangea Root

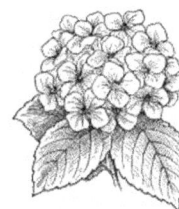

HYDRANGEA ROOT can be helpful for treating the bladder. It treats infections and stones in the bladder, it treats bedwetting problems. Hydrangea Root may be taken in capsules. If it is taken as a tea, use ¼ teaspoon of Hydrangea herb powder to one cup of boiling water. Hydrangea may be taken as often as you feel the need. For treating the bladder it may be taken once or twice a day for two to five days or until desired results are reached. For some, once or twice a week can be helpful until desired results are reached. People with high blood pressure should not use this herb more than once a week.

Contains: sodium, sulphur, calcium, iron, potassium, and magnesium.

BLADDER

HERBS:

*Juniper

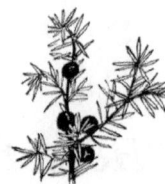

JUNIPER can be great for treating infections in the bladder. It treats kidney infections, increase the flow of urine from the bladder, treats diabetes and water retention. Juniper Berry will increase the production of insulin in the body. Do not take Juniper Berry if you suffer from kidney disease because it may over stimulate the kidneys and the adrenals. Juniper Berries may be taken in capsules, if it is taken as a tea, add ¼ teaspoon of Juniper Berries herb powder to one cup of boiling water. Juniper Berries may be taken as often as you feel the need for treating bladder infections. It may be taken once or twice a day, for two to five days, or until desired results are reached. For some, two or three times a week can offer excellent results.

Contains: sulphur, copper, a small amount of aluminum, and a high amount of vitamin C.

Lemon Grass

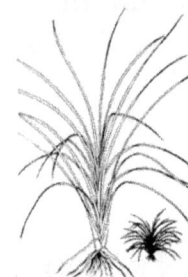

LEMON GRASS treats the bladder. It is an excellent blood cleanser and it treats kidneys, liver problems. It is excellent for treating fevers. It will help to treat nausea and vomiting. Lemon Grass may be taken in combination with other herbs. It will increase urination and help to treat internal parasites. Lemon Grass may be taken in capsules. If it is taken as a tea, use ¼ teaspoon of Lemon Grass herb powder to one cup of boiling water. Lemon Grass may be taken as often as you feel the need. For treating the bladder it may be taken once a day for two to five days or until desired results are reached. For some, once or twice a week can give good results.

Contains: calcium, iron, magnesium, manganese, phosphorus, potassium, selenium, zinc, Lemon Grass is high in vitamins A and C.

BLADDER

HERBS:

*Marshmallow

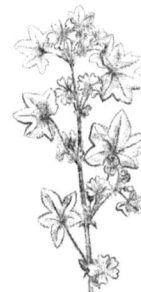

MARSHMALLOW will do wonders for the bladder. It treats the kidneys, and an inflamed urinary tract. Marshmallow will assist with treating painful urination. Mixed with Juniper Berries, Marshmallow works very well for treating blood in the urine. It removes kidney stones and gravel. Marshmallow is excellent for treating inflammation in the lungs. **Marshmallow may elevate blood pressure for some people when taken excessively.** It may be taken in capsules. If it is taken as a tea, use ¼ teaspoon of Marshmallow herb powder to one cup of boiling water. Marshmallow may be taken as often as you feel the need. For treating chronic bladder problems it may be taken two or three times a day for two to five days, or until the desired results are reached. For some two or three times a week will give treatment. You may only need to use this herb once for your bladder problems. Do not confuse Marshmallow herb with the candy like marshmallow found in the food section of the market.

Contains: sodium, iodine, B complex, pantothenic acid, and is high in calcium, zinc, and iron.

Oatstraw

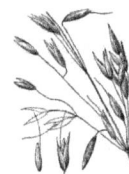

OATSTRAW relieves spasms in the bladder. It improves urinary organs. It treats kidney and liver problems. It helps to lower blood pressure and cholesterol. If one is recovering from an illness or drug withdrawals, this herb will help with recovery. Oatstraw can be helpful for treating thyroid and estrogen deficiency. Oatstraw stimulates the appetite Oatstraw should be taken at bedtime. Oatstraw may be taken in capsules. If it is taken as a tea, use ¼ teaspoon of Oatstraw herb powder to one cup of boiling water. Oatstraw may be taken as often as you feel the need. For treating chronic bladder problems it may be taken once or twice a day for two to seven days or until the desired results are reached. For some once or twice a week can offer results.

BLADDER

HERBS:

Contains: vitamins A, B1, B2, and E.

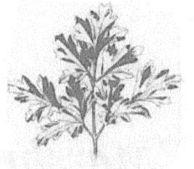

*Parsley

PARSLEY is a good herb to start with for treating the bladder. It treats kidney infections, painful urination, it can be helpful for treating incomplete urination. Parsley will increase low blood sugar. When this herb is used in large amounts for a long period it will sweeten the breath. Use this herb in moderation during pregnancy it will induce labor pains; however, after birth it will dry up mother's milk during the weaning period. Use ¼ teaspoons of Parsley herb powder to one cup of boiling water. Parsley may be taken as often as you feel the need. For bladder problems it may be taken once or twice a day until desired results are reached.

Herbs for your blood type: Parsley is highly beneficial for blood type O and B. It is neutral for people with blood type A and AB.

Contains: vitamins A, B, and C, chlorophyll, iron, potassium, calcium, cobalt, copper, riboflavin, silicon sodium, sulphur, and thiamine

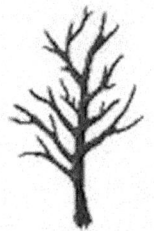

*Peach Bark

PEACH BARK relieves inflammation in the bladder. It treats the kidneys, burning in the urine, and it stimulates the flow of urine. It helps to relieve gas and colic, and treats the mucus membrane. **Pregnant women should not take Peach Bark, it can cause miscarriage.** Peach Bark can be taken in capsules. If it is taken as a tea, use ¼ teaspoon of Peach Bark herb powder to one cup of boiling water. Peach Bark may be taken as often as you feel the need. For chronic bladder problems it may be taken once or twice a day for two to seven days or until desired results are reached. For some, once or twice a week can be beneficial.

BLADDER

HERBS:

Plantain

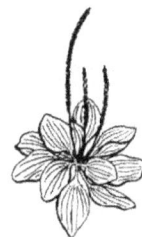

PLANTAIN is an excellent remedy for treating pain in the bladder. It treats kidney problems and eases the pain. Plantain herb powder will suppress the appetite and it lowers cholesterol. Plantain may be taken in capsules. If it is taken as a tea, use ¼ teaspoon of Plantain herb powder to one cup of boiling water. Plantain may be taken as often as you feel the need. For chronic bladder problems it may be taken once or twice a day for two to five days or until desired results are reached. For some, once or twice a week can be beneficial.

Contains: a high amount of vitamins C and K, calcium, sulphur, and potassium. Plantain is high in minerals.

*Queen of The Meadow

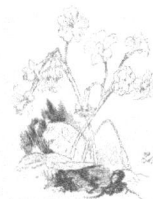

QUEEN OF THE MEADOW will be great for treating the bladder. It treats infections and stones in the bladder. It is excellent for treating urinary problems. It treats prostate and uterine disease, gravel and kidney infections. It will allow a very easy urine flow, especially if there is a chronic problem. It may be taken in capsules. If it is taken as a tea, use ¼ teaspoon of Queen of The Meadow herb powder to one cup of boiling water. Queen of the Meadow may be taken as often as you feel the need. For chronic bladder problems it may be taken once or twice a day for two to seven days or until desired results are reached. For some, once or twice a week can be beneficial.

Contains: vitamins A, C, and D.

79

BLADDER

HERBS:

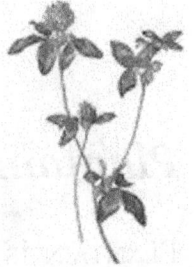

*Red Clover

RED CLOVER treats spasms in the bladder. It treats kidney and urinary problems, cancer, leukemia and vaginal irritation. Red Clover may be taken in capsules. If it is taken as a tea, use ¼ teaspoon of Red Clover herb powder to one cup of boiling water. Red Clover may be taken as often as you feel the need. For treating chronic bladder irritations it may be taken once a day for two to five days or until desired results are reached. For some, once a week can be beneficial.

Contains: vitamins A, B complex, calcium, sodium, nickel, manganese, and tin, Red Clover is high in iron and calcium.

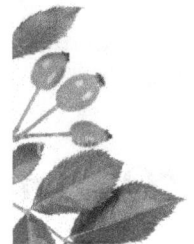

Rose Hips

ROSE HIPS will strengthen and prevent infections in the bladder. It treats the kidneys and has cancer-fighting powers. For people that are allergic to citrus, Rose Hips is an excellent alternative to vitamin C. Rose Hips may be taken in capsules. If it is taken as a tea, use ¼ teaspoon of Rose Hips herb powder to one cup of boiling water. Rose Hips may be taken as often as you feel the need. For bladder infections it may be taken once or twice a day for two to five days or until desired results are reached. For some, once or twice a week will be helpful.

Herbs for your Blood type: Rose Hips is highly beneficial for people with blood type O, A, B, and AB.

Contains: iron, sodium, sulphur, potassium, niacin, vitamins A, B complex, C, and E.

BLADDER

HERBS:

Sage

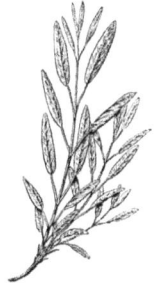

SAGE will strengthen and clear up infections in the bladder. It treats kidney and liver problems. Sage will dry up saliva, perspiration, and mother's milk. It may be taken in capsules. If it is taken as a tea, use ¼ teaspoon of Sage herb powder to one cup of boiling water. Sage may be taken as often as you feel the need. For treating the bladder it may be taken once or twice a day for two to five days or until desired results are reached. For some, once or twice a week can be helpful. People with high blood pressure should not take this herb more than once a week.

Herbs for your Blood type: Sage is highly beneficial for people with blood type B. It is neutral for people with blood type O, A, and AB.

Contains: sodium, sulphur, vitamins A, B complex, and C.

Saw Palmetto

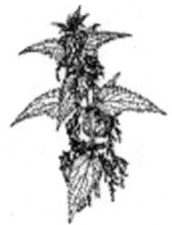

SAW PALMETTO can helpful with treating the bladder. It treats kidney diseases. Saw Palmetto stimulates the appetite and quiets the nerves. It increases blood flow to the sexual organs for both male and female. Saw Palmetto treats men that suffer from impotence due to alcohol disease. It is best used in conjunction with other herbs. Saw Palmetto may be taken in capsules. If it is taken as a tea, use ¼ teaspoon of Saw palmetto herb powder to one cup of boiling water. Saw Palmetto may be taken as often as you feel the need. For treating the bladder it may be taken once or twice a day for two to seven days or until desired results are reached. For some, once or twice a week can be helpful.

BLADDER

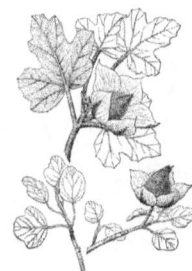

Slippery Elm

SLIPPERY ELM will assist with treating the bladder. It treats the kidneys and gives a smooth bowel elimination as well. Slippery Elm should be taken in capsules because it will not dissolve in liquid. Slippery Elm may be taken as often as you feel the need. For bladder/ problems it may be taken once a day for two to five days, or until desired results are reached. For some, once or twice a week can be beneficial. .

Herbs for your Blood type: Slippery Elm is highly beneficial for people with blood type O, and blood type A. It is neutral with blood type B and AB.

Contains: iron, sodium, iodine, zinc, copper, potassium, and vitamins K and E.

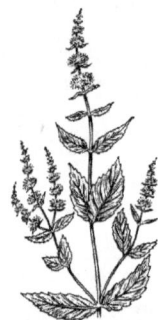

Spearmint

SPEARMINT can be helpful for the bladder. It treats painful burning urination, and vomiting. It is an excellent herb to use for the sickest person and gentle enough for babies with colic. Spearmint can be taken in capsules. If it is taken as a tea, use ¼ teaspoon of Spearmint herb powder to one cup of boiling water. Spearmint may be taken as often as you feel the need. For treating the bladder it may be taken once or twice a day for two to seven days or until desired results are reached. For some once or twice a week can be helpful.

Herbs for your Blood type: Spearmint is neutral for people with blood type O, A, B and AB.

Contains: calcium, iron, sulphur, iodine, potassium, magnesium, vitamin A, C, and B complex.

BLADDER

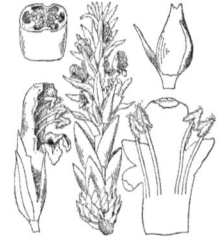

Squaw Vine

Squaw Vine will assist with treating the bladder. It treats urinary disease and it promotes urination. Squaw Vine treats bleeding and uterine disorders. Use Squaw Vine in combination with other herbs. It will help with water retention. Squaw Vine may be taken in capsules. If it is taken as a tea, use ¼ teaspoon of the combined herbs to one cup of boiling water. Square Vine may be taken once or twice a week until the desired results are reached.

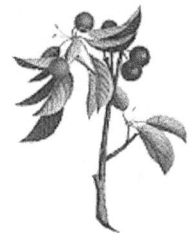

*Uva Ursi

Uva Ursi treats chronic problems in the bladder. It clears up blood in the urine. It treats inflammation in the urinary tract and it is a tonic for the walls of the bladder, and promotes bladder control; Uva Ursi increases the flow of urine and acts as a disinfectant. Uva Ursi will turn the urine a dark green do not panic it is normal while taking this herb. This herb treats bedwetting. Use a small amount in the beginning and increase the amount as necessary. **Large quantities of Uva Ursi during pregnancy could possibly be harmful to the fetus by decreasing circulation to it.** Uva Ursi may be taken in capsules. If it is taken as a tea, use 1/8th teaspoon or less of Uva Ursi herb powder to one cup of boiling water. Uva Ursi may be taken as often as you feel the need. For chronic bladder problems it may be taken once or twice a day for two to five days or until desired results are reached. For some, two or three times a week can be beneficial.

Contains: iron, manganese, trace minerals, and vitamin A.

BLADDER

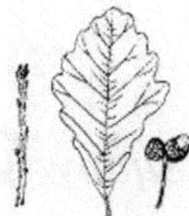

White Oak Bark

WHITE OAK BARK will help with treating infections in the bladder. It treats an ulcerated bladder. White Oak Bark will increase urine flow, and give support to the bladder. It treats PMS and it can be useful for treating external and internal bleeding. White Oak Bark **may elevate blood pressure for some people when taken excessively**. It should be taken in combination with Burdock or Kelp, but not necessary. White Oak Bark may be taken in capsules. If it is taken as a tea, use ¼ teaspoon of White Oak Bark herb powder to one cup of boiling water. White Oak Bark may be taken as often as you feel the need. For infections in the bladder it may be taken two or three times a day, for three to seven days, or until desired results are reached. For some, once or twice a week can be helpful.

Contains: sodium, cobalt, lead, iodine, potassium, calcium, sulphur, and vitamin B12.

BLEEDING

Agrimony

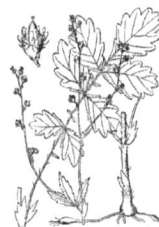

AGRIMONY is helpful for treating uterine bleeding. It has also been known to treat bleeding wounds. For treating wounds it is best used as a poultice. Apply the poultice after cleaning the wound. Agrimony is high in nutrients and is a tonic. Agrimony is a pleasant tasting herb and it may be taken in capsules. If it is taken as a tea, use ¼ teaspoon of Agrimony herb powder to one cup of boiling water. Agrimony may be taken as often as you feel the need. For bleeding it may be taken once or twice a day, for two to five days, or until desired results are reached. A poultice may be applied as often as desired.

Contains: iron, niacin, vitamin K, and B3.

*Alfafa

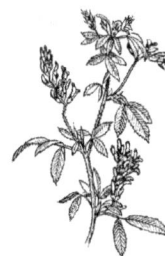

ALFALFA is especially good for stopping bleeding. It stops hemorrhages and nose bleeds. It is beneficial as a colon cancer preventative. Alfalfa will stimulate the appetite, and treat acidity in the stomach. It is a pleasant tasting herb and it may be taken in capsules, if it is taken as a tea, use ¼ teaspoon of Alfalfa herb powder to one cup of boiling water. Alfalfa may be taken as often as you feel the need. For hemorrhaging it may be taken two or three times a day until desired results are reached. For some, once or twice a week can be a good prevention.

Herbs for your blood type: Alfalfa is highly beneficial for people with blood type A. It is neutral for people with blood type B and AB. People with blood type O should avoid this herb it will cause excessive blood thinning for them.

BLEEDING

HERBS:

Contains: Vitamins A, D, and K, iron, potassium, and phosphorus. Alfalfa is very high in calcium and chlorophyll.

*Aloe

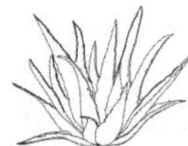

ALOE leaf is excellent for stopping bleeding. It treats minor cuts, burns and insect bites. It will reduce the likelihood of infection. Use the gel of the leaf and rub it on the affected area. Wash the Aloe leaf with cold water, split the leaf in half and use the bleeding gel inside the leaf on the wound. Aloe may be taken as often as you feel the need. For bleeding it may be taken once or twice a day for desired results.

   Herbs for your blood type: Aloe is highly beneficial for people with blood type A. People with blood type O, B, or AB should avoid this herb" internally. However, used externally, Aloe leaf is great for the skin of all blood types.

Contains: Calcium, iron, sodium, potassium, magnesium, lecithin, and zinc.

*Bayberry

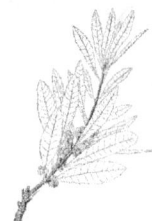

BAYBERRY can be excellent for treating excessive vaginal bleeding. It will also help with infections of wounds. It may be used as a poultice externally and taken internally at the same time. Bayberry may be taken in capsules. If it is taken as a tea, use ¼ teaspoon of Bayberry herb powder to one cup of boiling water. Bayberry may be taken as often as you feel the need. For profuse bleeding it may be taken two or three times a day for two to five days, or until desired result are reached. For some it may only need to be used once for desired results.

Contains: potassium, sodium, niacin, calcium, magnesium, manganese, silicon, zinc, vitamins B1, B2, and C.

BLEEDING

HERBS:

Birch

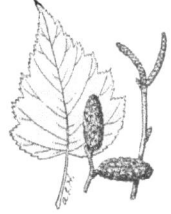

BIRCH will assist with treating bleeding. It treats bleeding gums and pyorrhea of the gums. Use it as a gargle. When taken internally it treats cancer, pain, and urinary problems. It is best taken at bedtime due to its mild sedative properties. Birch may be taken in capsules. If it is taken as a tea, use ¼ teaspoon of Birch herb powder to one cup of boiling water. Birch may be taken as often as you feel the need. For bleedings it may be taken once or twice a day until desired results are reached. It may only be used once for some.

Contains: copper, sodium, calcium, iron, magnesium, potassium, silicon, and vitamins A, B1, B2, C, and E.

*Bistort

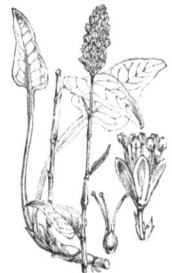

BISTORT is an excellent antiseptic to use for bleeding. It treats both externally and internally. Use it externally to wash wounds. Bistort may be used as a mouthwash for bleeding gums. When used internally it may be taken in capsules, if it is taken as a tea, use ¼ teaspoon of Bistort herb powder to one cup of boiling water. Bistort may be taken as often as you feel the need. For bleeding it may be taken once or twice a day until desired results are reached.

Contains: Vitamins A and B complex, and is very high in vitamin C.

BLEEDING

HERBS:

Blackberry

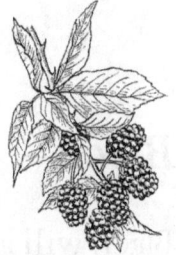

BLACKBERRY can be good for treating excessive vaginal bleeding. It treats bleeding of the gums, sinus problems and vomiting. Blackberry may be taken in capsules. If it is taken as a tea, use ¼ teaspoon of blackberry herb powder to one cup of boiling water. Blackberry may be taken as often as you feel the need. For bleeding it may be taken once or twice a day until desired results are reached.

   Herbs for your blood type: Blackberry is highly beneficial for people with blood type A. It is neutral for people with blood type B and AB. People with blood type O should avoid this herb.

*Buckthorn

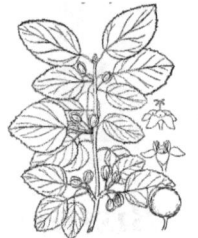

BUCKTHORN can be excellent for stopping bleeding. It can be used to treat cancer, and chronic constipation. It treats lead poisoning and liver problems. Buckthorn may be used externally, as well as internally, for bleeding. Buckthorn will cause griping and cramps when used excessively. Buckthorn may be taken in capsules. If it is taken as a tea, use ¼ teaspoon of Buckthorn herb powder to one cup of boiling water. Buckthorn may be taken as often as you feel the need. For treating bleeding it may be taken once or twice a day, for two to five days, or until desired results are reached.

Contains vitamin C.

BLEEDING

HERBS:

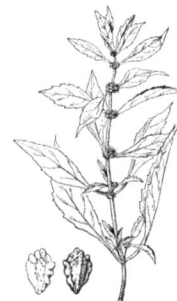

Bugleweed

BUGLEWEED will help to stop excessive menstrual bleeding. It treats other internal bleeding, especially the lungs. It calms the nerves, and the heart, and it will lower the pulse and stabilize an irregular heartbeat. Pregnant and nursing women should not use Bugleweed. Bugleweed may be taken in capsules. If it is taken as a tea, use ¼ teaspoon of Bugleweed herb powder to one cup of boiling water. Bugleweed may be taken as often as you feel the need. For treating bleeding it may be taken once or twice a day, for two to five days, or until desired results are reached.

Contains Tannin.

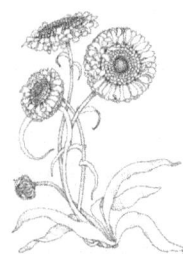

Calendula

CALENDULA will assist with treating bleeding. It treat cuts when applied as a poultice. It is a strong antiseptic with a natural content of iodine. Calendula is known for treating tetanus and gangrene. It will work faster when taken internally and externally together. If it is taken internally as a tea, use ¼ teaspoon of Calendula herb powder to one cup of boiling water. Calendula may be taken as often as you feel the need. For bleeding it may be taken internally once or twice a day until desired results are reached. As a poultice it may applied to the wound as often as needed.

BLEEDING

HERBS:

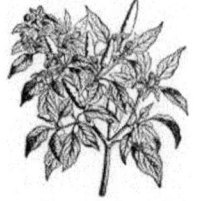

*Capsicum/Cayenne

CAPSICUM/CAYENNE is good for treating bleeding. It treats both internal and external bleeding. When used externally as a poultice it will purify wounds. Capsicum/Cayenne is a peppery herb and may be kept in the kitchen as a spice. When Capsicum/Cayenne is taken internally it can be used in conjunction with other herbs. It may be taken in capsules. When it is taken as a tea, use 1/8 teaspoon or less of Capsicum/Cayenne herb powder to one cup of boiling water. Capsicum/Cayenne may be used as often as needed. For treating bleeding, it may be used once or twice a day, for two to three days, or until desired results are reached.

Herbs for your blood type: Capsicum/Cayenne is highly beneficial for people with blood type O. It is neutral for people with blood B and AB. People with blood type A should avoid the herb.

Contains: vitamins A and C, magnesium, and sulphur. Capsicum/Cayenne is very high in iron, potassium, and calcium.

Chickweed

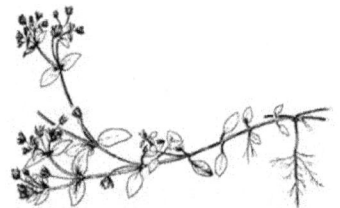

CHICKWEED will assist with treating bleeding. It treats internal and external bleeding. Chickweed powder may be mixed with water. Apply the mixture to the wound. It treats blood poisoning, cancer tumors, and cholesterol. Chickweed suppresses the appetite. It can be used internally and externally at the same time. It may be taken in capsules. If it is taken as a tea, use ¼ teaspoon of Chickweed herb powder to one cup of boiling water. Chickweed may be taken as often as you feel the need. For internal bleeding it may be taken once or twice a day, for two to three days, or until desired results are reached. Externally it may be applied as often as necessary.

Herbs for your blood type: Chickweed is highly beneficial for people with blood type O. It is neutral for people with blood type A, B, and AB.

BLEEDING

Comfrey

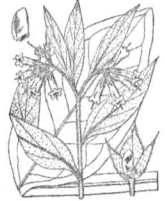

COMFREY will help to stop bleeding. It will treat bleeding in the bowels. It treats hemorrhaging, piles, blood in the urine, and stomach problems. Comfrey extract liquid can be poured directly onto a wound to help avoid the need for stitches. It treats cancer, stimulates new cell growth and provides general healing. Comfrey may be taken in capsules, if it is taken as a tea use ¼ teaspoon of Comfrey herb powder to one cup of boiling water. Comfrey may be taken as often as you feel the need. For treating internal bleeding it may be taken once or twice a day, for two to seven days, or until desired results are reached. Comfrey may only need to be taken once or twice for desired results.

Contains: vitamins A, C, iron, sulphur, copper, zinc, magnesium, and Comfrey is very high in calcium, potassium, and protein.

Cramp Bark

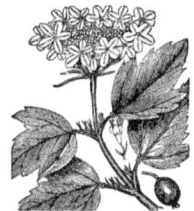

CRAMP BARK will assist with treating bleeding. It treats bleeding ulcers and menstrual cramps. Some herbalists recommend this herb to prevent miscarriage and ovarian problems. Cramp Bark may be taken in capsules. If it is taken as a tea, use ¼ teaspoon of Cramp Bark herb powder to one cup of boiling water. Cramp Bark may be taken as often as you feel the need. For bleeding it may be taken once or twice a day, for two to five days, or until desired results are reached. For some, once or twice may be all that is needed for results.

Contains: calcium, potassium, and magnesium and is very high in vitamins C, and K.

BLEEDING

HERBS:

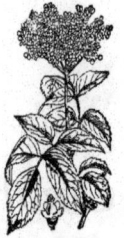

*Dong Quai

DONG QUAI will treat any type of internal bleeding. It will treat internal bleeding, Dong Quai purifies the blood, treats cancer, menstrual problems, nervousness, and a prolapsed uterus. It will lubricate the intestines as it heals. It is useful for pregnant mothers. Dong Quai may be taken in capsules, if it is taken as a tea, use ¼ teaspoon of Dong Quai herb powder to one cup of boiling water. Dong Quai may be taken as often as you feel the need. For bleeding it may be taken once or twice a day, for two to five days, or until desired results are reached. For some, once or twice a week can be helpful for prevention.

   Herbs for your blood type: Dong Quai is neutral for people with blood type O, A, B and AB.

Contains: vitamins A, B12, and E.

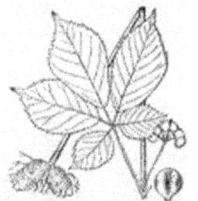

Ginseng/Panax

GINSENG/PANAX will be helpful to stop internal bleeding. It is often used for treating cancer, depression, and it offers longevity and vitality. Ginseng/Panax will increase the appetite. Long-term regular use is not recommended for women, as it will produce testosterone, which will increase hormones. One week on and three weeks off will do fine for women. This herb will benefit men on long-term use just great! Ginseng/Panax is better prepared in glass cookware. Metal pots will reduce the strength. It may be taken in capsules, if it is taken as a tea use ¼ teaspoon of Ginseng/Panax herb powder to one cup of boiling water. Ginseng/Panax may be taken as often as you feel the need. For internal bleeding it may be taken once or twice a day, for two to five days, or until desired results are reached. For some, once or twice a week can be beneficial for prevention.

   Herbs for your blood type: Ginseng is highly beneficial for Blood types O, A, B, and AB.

BLEEDING

HERBS:

*Juniper

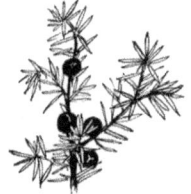

JUNIPER is great for stopping internal bleeding. When used externally, it may be applied directly to the wound as a poultice. It treats arthritis, and contagious diseases. Juniper is not recommended for pregnant women. Juniper produces natural insulin in the body. Juniper may be taken in capsules. If it is taken as a tea, use ¼ teaspoon of Juniper herb powder to one cup of boiling water. Juniper may be taken as often as you feel the need. For bleeding it may be taken once or twice a day, for two to five days, or until desired results are reached. For some, once or twice a week can be beneficial for prevention.

Contains: sulphur, copper, a small amount of aluminum, and is high in vitamin C.

*Marshmallow

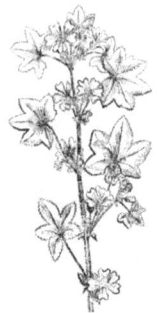

MARSHMALLOW is especially good for treating bleeding. It treats vaginal and urinary bleeding. It treats nervous problems, pneumonia, and whooping cough. Marshmallow may be taken in capsules. If it is taken as a tea, use ¼ teaspoon of Marshmallow herb powder to one cup of boiling water. Marshmallow may be taken as often as you feel the need. For bleeding it may be taken once or twice a day, for two to five days, or until desired results are reached. **Marshmallow may elevate blood pressure for some people when taken excessively.** People with high blood pressure should not use Marshmallow more than once a week.

Do not confuse Marshmallow herb with the candy like marshmallow found in the food section of the market.

Contains: sodium, iodine, B complex, and pantothenic acid, and is high in calcium, zinc, and iron.

BLEEDING

*Mullein

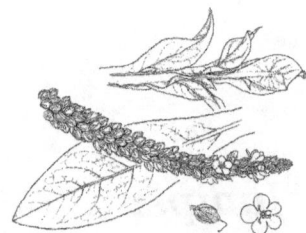

MULLEIN is excellent for treating bleeding. It treats bleeding in the bowels. It treats the lungs, allergies, asthma, emphysema, and swollen glands **Mullein is best taken at bedtime because it will cause sleepiness.** It may be taken in capsules. If it is taken as a tea, use ¼ teaspoon of Mullein herb powder to one cup of boiling water. Mullein may be taken as often as you feel the need. For treating bleeding bowels it may be taken two or three times a day, for three to five days, or until desired results are reached. You may only need to use Mullein once.

Herbs for your blood type: Mullein is neutral for people with blood type O, and A. People with Blood type B and AB should avoid this herb.

Contains: magnesium, potassium, and sulphur. Mullein is very high in iron.

*Nettle

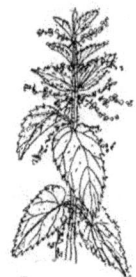

NETTLE is excellent for treating excessive bleeding. It treats menstrual bleeding; and other internal bleeding. It treats nosebleeds, dysentery, infections, and inflamed kidneys. The hair will receive benefits from Nettle as well. Nettle may be taken in capsules. If it is taken as a tea, use ¼ teaspoon of Nettle herb powder to one cup of boiling water. Nettle may be taken as often as you feel the need. For excessive bleeding it may be taken two or three times a day for two to five days, or until desired results are reached.

Contains: vitamins A, C, D, E, F, and P, copper, potassium, sodium, calcium, chlorophyll, sulphur, silicon, protein, zinc, and is high in iron and minerals.

BLEEDING

Periwinkle

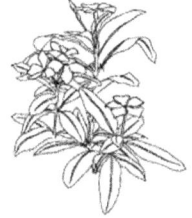

PERIWINKLE is an ideal herb to treat nose bleeding. It also stops internal bleeding of hemorrhoids. Periwinkle has been known to stop an excess flow of blood. Periwinkle will protect brain cells and increase oxygen flow to the brain. It helps to reduce brain injury after strokes. Periwinkle is also a sedative. **Do not over use Periwinkle.** It may be taken in capsules. If it is taken as a tea, use ¼ teaspoon of Periwinkle herb powder to one cup of boiling water. Periwinkle should be used with caution. For bleeding problems it may be taken once a day for two days.

*Plantain

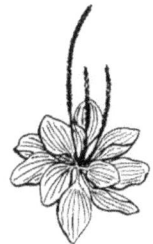

PLANTAIN can be great for treating internal bleeding. It treats open sores, chronic burns, and wounds. It may be used as a poultice for external bleeding. Plantain will suppress the appetite and it lowers cholesterol. It may be taken in capsules. If it is taken as a tea, use ¼ teaspoon of Plantain herb powder to one cup of boiling water. Plantain may be taken as often as you feel the need, for bleeding it may be taken once or twice a day for two to five days, or until desired results are reached.

Contains: a high amount of vitamins C and K, calcium, sulphur, potassium, and is high in minerals.

BLEEDING
---

*Shepard's Purse

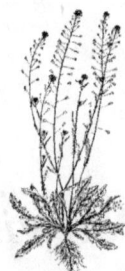

SHEPHERD'S PURSE will control internal bleeding. It will coagulate the blood. Shepherd's Purse stops excessive menstruation flow and bloody urine. It is an astringent and can be effective in regulating blood pressure. It lowers high blood pressure and raises low blood pressure. Shepherd's Purse may be taken in capsules. If it is taken as a tea, use ¼ teaspoon of Shepherd's Purse herb powder to one cup of boiling water. Shepherd's Purse may be taken as often as you feel the need. For bleeding, it can be taken once or twice a day, for two to five days, or until desired results are reached.

Herbs for your blood type: Shepherd's Purse is neutral for people with blood type A. People with blood type O, B and AB should avoid this herb.

Contains: sodium, calcium, potassium, zinc, sulphur, magnesium, vitamins E and K, and it is very high in vitamin C.

Squaw Vine

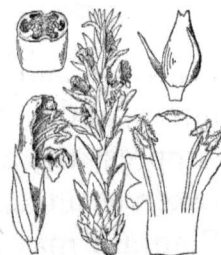

SQUAW VINE will help with bleeding. It treats hemorrhoids. It treats painful and irregular menstrual problems. Squaw Vine treats water retention and urinary problems. Squaw Vine may be taken in capsules. If it is taken as a tea, use ¼ teaspoon of Squaw Vine herb powder to one cup of boiling water. Squaw Vine may be taken as often as you feel the need. For internal bleeding it may be taken once or twice a day, for two to five days, or until desired results are reached.

BLEEDING

White Oak Bark

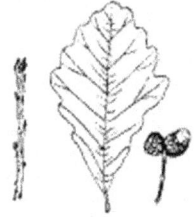

WHITE OAK BARK will treat excessive menstrual bleeding; it treats stomach, liver, and bowel bleeding. It treats a prolapsed uterus, prostate problems, and nausea. White Oak Bark may be taken in capsules. If it is taken as a tea, use ¼ teaspoon of White Oak Bark herb powder to one cup of boiling water. White Oak Bark may be taken as often as you feel the need. For bleeding it may be taken two or three times a day for two to five days, or until desired results are reached.

Contains: sodium, cobalt, lead, iodine, potassium, calcium, sulphur, and vitamin B12.

BLOOD PURIFIERS

Alfafa

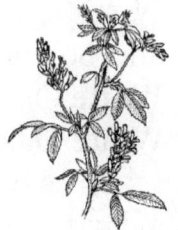

ALFALFA is great for purifying the blood. It treats allergies, asthma, and blood clotting. It treats fatigue and stimulates the appetite. It treats acidity. Alfalfa may be taken in capsules. If it is taken as a tea, use ¼ teaspoon of Alfalfa herb powder to one cup of boiling water. Alfalfa may be taken as often as you feel the need. For purifying the blood it may be taken once or twice a day, for three to five days, or until desired results are reached. For some, two or three times a week can be beneficial.

Herbs for your blood type: Alfalfa is highly beneficial for people with blood type A. It is neutral for people with blood type B and AB. People with blood type O should avoid this herb it will cause excessive blood thinning for them.

Contains: vitamins A, B complex, D, E, and K, iron, potassium, magnesium, protein, sodium, sulfur, and phosphorus. Alfalfa is very high in calcium, chlorophyll, and vitamin B12.

Aloe

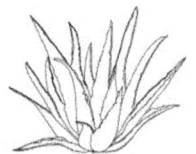

ALOE is excellent for purifying and cleaning the blood. It cleans the colon, treats AIDS, and allergies. Aloe treats bleeding, and radiation burns. It is a buffer for the HIV virus. Aloe may be taken in capsules. If it is taken as a tea, use ¼ teaspoon of Aloe herb powder to one cup of boiling water. Aloe may be taken as often as you feel the need. For cleaning chronic blood problems it may be taken once daily until desired results are reached.

BLOOD PURIFIERS

HERBS:

Herbs for your blood type: Aloe is highly beneficial for people of blood type A. People with blood type O, B, and AB should avoid this herb internally.

Contains: calcium, iron, sodium, potassium, magnesium, lecithin, and zinc.

*Barberry

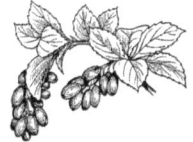

BARBERRY is excellent for purifying the blood. Before any illness can be treated successfully, the blood must be purified. Barberry cleans the blood; it treats arthritis, bladder infections, and bronchitis. Barberry should not be used excessively it may cause depression. It may be taken in capsules. If it is taken as a tea, use ¼ teaspoon of Barberry herb powder to one cup of boiling water. Barberry may be taken as often as you feel the need. For purifying chronic blood problems it may be taken two or three times a day, for two to five days, or until desired results are reached. For some once or twice a week can be helpful.

Contains: iron, manganese, phosphorus, and vitamin C.

*Black Cohosh

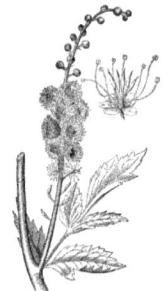

BLACK COHOSH is a blood cleanser and blood purifier. It should not be overlooked. It treats fevers, and inflammation. It's great for treating hot flashes, kidney, and lung problems. It treats poison bites, rheumatism, and St. Vitus' Dance. **Black Cohosh should be used in small amounts or it can cause a headache.** Black Cohosh lowers the heart rate slightly and increases the pulse rate. **Black Cohosh will induce labor when pregnant.** Black Cohosh should be used in combination with other herbs. Black Cohosh may be taken in capsules. When it is taken as a tea, use 1/8th teaspoon or less of Black Cohosh herb powder to one cup of boiling water. Black Cohosh may be taken as often as you feel the need. For purifying chronic blood problems it may be taken once or twice a day until desired results are reached. For some, once or twice a week should give results in a short period.

BLOOD PURIFIERS

HERBS:

Contains: calcium, potassium, iron, magnesium, manganese, niacin, phosphorus, selenium, silicon, sodium, sulphur, vitamins A, B1, B2, C, K, and F, and zinc.

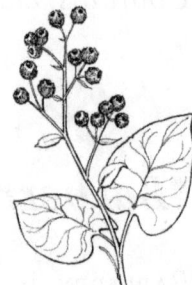

*Burdock

BURDOCK is an excellent blood purifier. It cleans the blood like no other herb. It treats arthritis, cancer, boils, constipation, fevers, gout, and rheumatism. Burdock will increase urine flow. Do not use an excessive amount of Burdock at one time; it may cause vomiting. Burdock is a pleasant tasting herb, and may be taken in capsules. If it is taken as a tea, use ¼ teaspoon of Burdock herb powder to one cup of boiling water. Burdock may be taken as often as you feel the need. For purifying chronic blood problems it may be taken once or twice a day, for three to seven days, or until desired results are reached. For some once or twice a week can be beneficial for two to three weeks.

Herbs for your blood type: Burdock is highly beneficial for people with blood type A and AB. It is neutral for people with blood type B. People with blood type O should avoid this herb it will cause excessive blood thinning and excessive bleeding.

Contains: vitamins A, B complex, C, E, iron, zinc, and sulphur.

BLOOD PURIFIERS

HERBS:

*Chickweed

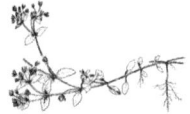

CHICKWEED is an excellent blood purifier. It removes poisons and plaque from the circulatory system. It treats cancer, cellulite, cholesterol, and gout. Chickweed is great for reducing and removing tumors, and it helps to reduce weight. It may be taken in capsules. If it is taken as a tea, use ¼ teaspoon of Chickweed herb powder to one cup of boiling water. Chickweed may be taken as often as you feel the need. For purifying chronic blood problems it may be taken once or twice a day, for two to seven days, or until desired results are reached. For some once or twice a week can be beneficial for two to three weeks.

Herbs for your blood type: Chickweed is highly beneficial for people with blood type O. It is neutral for people with blood type A, B, and AB.

Contains: iron, vitamins C, D, B complex, sodium, and zinc.

*Echinacea

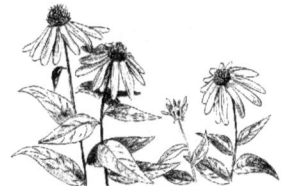

ECHINACEA is an excellent blood purifier. It expels toxins, poisons, and cleanses the blood. Echinacea will increase white blood cells. It treats infections, and skin problems. Echinacea may be taken in capsules. If it is taken as a tea, use ¼ teaspoon of Echinacea herb powder to one cup of boiling water. Echinacea may be taken as often as you feel the need. For purifying chronic blood problems it may be taken once or twice a day, for two to five days, or until desired results are reached. For some once or twice a week can be beneficial in a short period.

Herbs for your blood type: Echinacea is highly beneficial for people with blood type A and AB. It is neutral for people with blood type B. People with blood type O should avoid this herb; it will cause excessive blood thinning for them.

Contains: vitamins A, C, and E, iron, iodine, copper, sulphur, and potassium.

BLOOD PURIFIERS

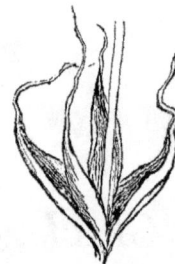

*Holy Thistle

HOLY THISTLE is a great blood purifier. It is also known as Holy Thistle. It treats poor circulation and removes calcium deposits from the blood. It increases oxygen to the brain. It treats cancer and strengthens the lungs. Holy Thistle may be taken in capsules. If it is taken as a tea, use ¼ teaspoon of Holy Thistle herb powder to one cup of boiling water. Holy Thistle may be taken as often as you feel the need. For purifying chronic blood problems it may be taken once or twice a day, for two to five days, or until desired results are reached. For some once or twice a week can be beneficial for two to three weeks.

Contains: B complex, calcium, iron, manganese, and potassium.

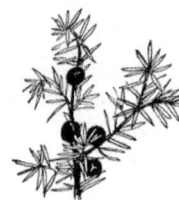

Juniper

JUNIPER will help to purify the blood; it removes waste from the bloodstream, treats bladder problems, and excessive bleeding. It's great for treating infections and urinary problems. Pregnant women should not take juniper. Juniper may be taken in capsules, if it is taken as a tea, use ¼ teaspoon of Juniper to one cup of boiling water. Juniper may be taken as often as you feel the need. For purifying the blood it may be taken once or twice a day, for two to five days, or until desired results are reached. For some once or twice a week should give results in a short period.

Contains: sulphur, copper, a small amount of aluminum, and a high amount of vitamin C.

BLOOD PURIFIERS

HERBS:

*Oregon Grape

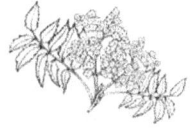

OREGON GRAPE is an excellent blood purifier. It treats acne, staph infections, and jaundice. Oregon Grape has a stimulating effect on the thyroid functions. It cleans the liver and improves function of the immune system. Oregon Grape stimulates the appetite. Oregon Grape is a bitter herb and it may be taken in capsules. If it is taken as a tea, use ¼ teaspoon of Oregon Grape herb powder to one cup of boiling water. Oregon Grape may be taken as often as you feel the need. For purifying chronic blood problems it may be taken once or twice a day, for two to seven days, or until desired results are reached. For some once or twice a week can be beneficial for two to three weeks.

Contains: sodium, zinc, manganese, copper, and silicon.

Prickly Ash

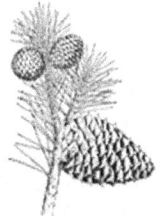

PRICKLY ASH will act as a blood purifier. It treats a wide variety of conditions, such as poor circulation, fevers, rheumatism and typhoid fever. Prickly Ash increases the flow of saliva, and treats mouth sores. Prickly Ash will increase circulation to the legs. It warms cold hands, cold feet, and cold legs. It may cause some people to become more sensitive to sunlight and burn more easily. It helps to treat yeast growth, and gonorrhea. Prickly Ash may be taken in capsules. If it is taken as a tea, use ¼ teaspoon of Prickly Ash herb powder to one cup of boiling water. Prickly Ash may be taken as often as you feel the need. For purifying the blood it may be taken once or twice a day, for three to seven days, or until desired results are reached. For some, once or twice a week can be helpful.

Contains tannins.

BLOOD PURIFIERS

HERBS:

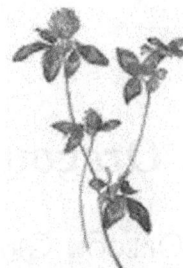

*Red Clover

RED CLOVER is an excellent blood purifier. It is an anti-cancer herb that treats leukemia, and liver problems. Red Clover may be taken in capsules. If it is taken as a tea, use ¼ teaspoon of Red Clover herb powder to one cup of boiling water. Red Clover may be taken as often as you feel the need. For purifying chronic blood problems it may be taken once a day, for two to five days, or until desired results are reached. For some, once or twice a year can be beneficial.

Contains: vitamins A, and B complex, calcium, sodium, nickel, manganese, tin, and is high in iron and calcium.

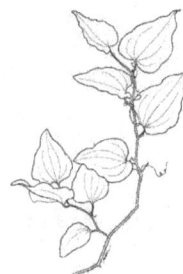

*Sarasparilla

SARSAPARILLA is at the top of the list for purifying the blood. It is a good anti-cancer herb. Some people use it as a natural steroid because it builds muscles. Sarsaparilla may elevate blood pressure for some people when taken excessively. If it must be taken, use only a pinch in combination with other herbs, making sure not to use it more than once a week. Sarsaparilla may be taken in capsules. If it is taken as a tea, use ¼ teaspoon of Sarsaparilla herb powder to one cup of boiling water. Sarsaparilla may be taken as often as you feel the need. For purifying the blood it may be taken once or twice a day, for two to seven days, or until desired results are reached. For some, once or twice a week can be beneficial.

Herbs for your blood type: Sarsaparilla is highly beneficial for people with blood type O. It is neutral for people with blood type A, B and AB.

Contains: iron, sodium, silicon, sulphur, zinc, iodine, copper, manganese, and vitamins A, B complex, C, and D.

BLOOD PURIFIERS

HERBS:

*Sassafras

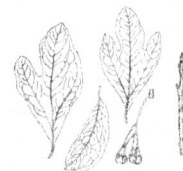

SASSAFRAS can be very beneficial for purifying the blood. It treats acne, skin diseases, obesity and water retention. Sassafras may be taken in capsules. If it is taken as a tea, use ¼ teaspoon of Sassafras herb powder to one cup of boiling water. Sassafras may be taken as often as you feel the need. For purifying chronic blood problems it may be taken once or twice a day, for two to seven days, or until desired results are reached. For some, once or twice a week can give results in a short period.

Contains: ascorbic acid, vitamin A, and is high in protein.

Wood Betony

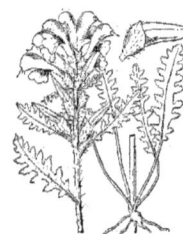

WOOD BETONY will clean impurities from the blood. It treats jaundice, migraine headaches, and liver problems. Wood Betony will increase the frequency of urination. It is soothing to children as well as adults. Wood Betony may be taken in capsules. If it is taken as a tea, use ¼ teaspoon of Wood Betony herb powder to one cup of boiling water. Wood Betony may be taken as often as you feel the need. For purifying the blood it may be taken once or twice a day until desired results are reached. For some, once or twice a week can give results in a short period.

Contains: vitamin C, manganese, and phosphorus.

BLOOD PURIFIERS

HERBS:

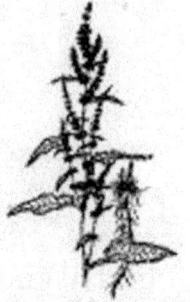

*Yellow Dock

YELLOW DOCK is one of the best-known blood purifiers. It cleanses the blood. It is excellent for cleansing the lymphatic system and treating anemia. It treats arthritis and cancer. Yellow Dock may be taken in capsules. If it is taken as a tea, use ¼ teaspoon of Yellow Dock herb powder to one cup of boiling water. Yellow Dock may be taken as often as you feel the need. For purifying the blood it may be taken once or twice a day, for three to seven days, or until desired results are reached. For some once or twice a week can be beneficial in a short period.

Herbs for your blood type: Yellow Dock is neutral for people with blood type B and AB. People with blood type O, and A should avoid this herb.

Contains: vitamins A, C, and nickel, and is very high in iron.

BRONCHITIS

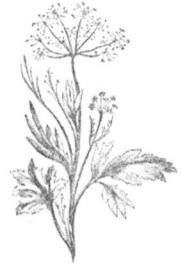

Anise

ANISE will assist with treating bronchitis. It treats asthma, cholera, emphysema and pneumonia. It stimulates the appetite. Use Anise in a vapor to help with breathing for bronchitis treatment. Anise is a stimulator for the heart, lungs, and brain. It produces high estrogen levels. It may be taken in capsules. When it is taken as a tea use ¼ teaspoon of Anise herb powder to one cup of boiling water. Anise may be taken as often as you feel the need. For bronchitis it may be used or taken once or twice a day for two to seven days, or until desired results are reached. For some, once or twice a week or periodically, as you feel the need can be helpful.

Contains iron, calcium, potassium, magnesium, and B vitamins.

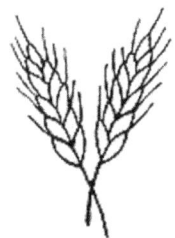

Barley Juice Powder

BARLEY JUICE POWDER can be helpful for treating bronchitis. It is excellent for treating arthritis and cancer. Barley Juice Powder will help to remove lead and mercury from the body. It may be taken in capsules. If it is taken as a tea, use ¼ teaspoon of Barley Powder to one cup of boiling water. Barley Juice Powder may be taken as often as you feel the need. For bronchitis it may be taken once or twice a day for two to five days, or until desired results are reached. For some, once or twice a week can be helpful.

Contains vitamins B1, B12, C, potassium, and iron. Barley Juice Powder is high in calcium.

BRONCHITIS

HERBS:

Bayberry

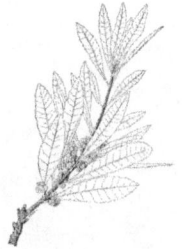

BAYBERRY is a stimulant that will help to treat bronchitis. It will help to remove mucus from the lungs. It treats cholera and it is a tonic that offers vitality to the body. Bayberry may be taken in capsules. If it is taken as a tea, use ¼ teaspoon of Bayberry herb powder to one cup of boiling water. Bayberry may be taken as often as you feel the need. For treating bronchitis it may be taken once or twice a day, for two to seven days, or until desired results are reached. For some, once or twice a week for two to three weeks, can help with prevention.

Contains: potassium, sodium, niacin, calcium, magnesium, manganese, silicon, zinc, vitamins B1, B2, and C.

*Black Cohosh

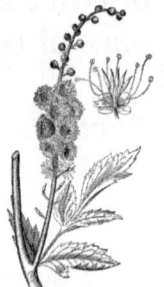

BLACK COHOSH can be great for treating chronic bronchitis. It cleans inflammation from the lungs, treats asthma, rheumatism and, tuberculosis. Black Cohosh should be used in small amounts or it can cause a headache. Black Cohosh lowers the heart rate slightly and will increase the pulse rate. It reduces hot flashes, and it is a sedative. Black Cohosh will induce labor when pregnant. It may be taken in capsules. If it is taken as a tea, use 1/8th teaspoon of Black Cohosh herb powder to one cup of boiling water. Black Cohosh may be taken as often as you feel the need. For chronic bronchitis it may be taken once or twice a day, for two to five days, or until desired results are reached. For some two or three times a week can be beneficial.

Contains: calcium, potassium, iron, magnesium, manganese, niacin, phosphorus, selenium, silicon, sodium, sulphur, zinc, vitamins A, B1, B2, C, K, and F.

BRONCHITIS

HERBS:

Blue Cohosh

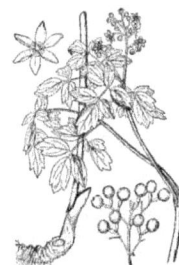

BLUE COHOSH will help to treat bronchitis. It treats dropsy, fits, hysteria, cleans the blood, and treats nervous disorders. Blue Cohosh will induce labor and should be used only in the ninth month of pregnancy. It is also a diuretic. Blue Cohosh is best used in combination with other herbs. Blue Cohosh may be taken in capsules. If it is taken as a tea, use 1/8th teaspoon or less of Blue Cohosh herb powder to one cup of boiling water. Blue Cohosh may be taken as often as you feel the need. For bronchitis it may be taken two or three times a day for two to five days, or until desired results are reached. For some two or three days a week will be helpful for two to three weeks.

Contains: vitamin E, calcium, B complex, potassium, phosphorus, and magnesium.

*Blue Vervain

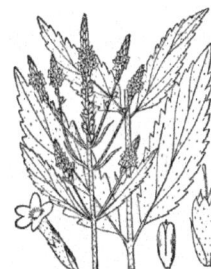

BLUE VERVAIN can be great for treating bronchitis. It offers a calm and tranquilizing effect to the system. It treats poor circulation, insomnia, toxic liver problems, and nervous disorders. Large amounts of Blue Vervain at once may cause vomiting. It may be taken in capsules. If it is taken as a tea, use ¼ teaspoon of Blue Vervain herb powder to one cup of boiling water. Blue Vervain may be taken as often as you feel the need. For chronic bronchitis it may be taken once or twice a day, for two to five days, or until the desired results are reached. For some two or three times a week will be beneficial.

Contains: vitamin C, calcium, manganese, and vitamin E.

BRONCHITIS

HERBS:

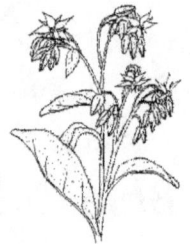

*Borage

BORAGE offers one of the best treatments for bronchitis. It treats inflammation of the eyes, strengthens the heart, and acts as a tonic for the entire body. Borage may be taken in capsules. If it is taken as a tea, use ¼ teaspoon of Borage herb powder to one cup of boiling water. Borage may be taken as often as you feel the need. For chronic bronchitis it may be taken two or three times a day until the desired results are reached. For some two or three times a week can be beneficial.

Contains: calcium and potassium.

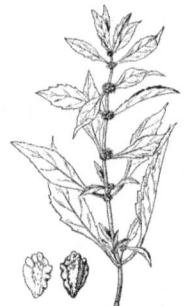

Bugleweed

BUGLEWEED can be useful for treating bronchitis. It reduces mucus from the body and eliminates coughs. It calms the nerves and the heart, it lowers the pulse and stabilizes an irregular heartbeat. Bugleweed may be taken in capsules. If it is taken as a tea, use ¼ teaspoon of Bugleweed herb powder to one cup of boiling water.

Bugleweed may be taken as often as you feel the need. For chronic bronchitis it may be taken once or twice a day, for two to five days, or until desired results are reached. For some two or three times a week can be useful.

BRONCHITIS

Burdock

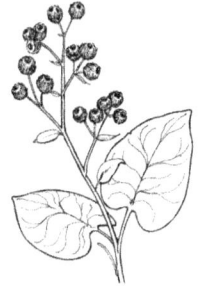

BURDOCK will assist with treating bronchitis. It helps to remove inflammation in the respiratory system. It treats the lungs, as well as gout. Burdock increases urine flow. Do not use an excessive amount of Burdock at one time; it may cause vomiting. It may be taken in capsules. If it is taken as a tea, use ¼ teaspoon of Burdock herb powder, to one cup of boiling water. Burdock may be taken as often as you feel the need. For chronic bronchitis it may be taken once or twice a day, for two to five days, or until desired results are reached. For some two or three times a week will give relief.

Herbs for your blood type: Burdock is highly beneficial for people with blood type A and AB. It is neutral for people with blood type B. People with blood type O should avoid this herb it will cause excessive blood thinning and excessive bleeding for them.

Contains: vitamins A, B complex, C, and E, iron, zinc, and sulphur.

Capsicum/Cayenne

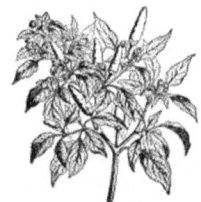

CAPSICUM/CAYENNE can be great for treating bronchitis. It treats fluid and inflammation in the lungs. It helps with treating the digestive system. It will increase perspiration and it stimulates circulation. Capsicum/Cayenne may be taken in capsules. If it is taken as a tea, use 1/8th teaspoon of capsicum/cayenne herb powder to one cup of boiling water. Capsicum/Cayenne may be taken as often as you feel the need. For treating chronic bronchitis it may be taken two or three times a day, for two to five days, or until desired results are reached. For some two or three times a week can help with prevention.

Herbs for your blood type: Capsicum/Cayenne is highly beneficial for people with blood type O. It is neutral for people with blood B and AB. People with blood type A should avoid this herb.

BRONCHITIS

HERBS:

Contains: vitamins A, C, magnesium, and sulphur. Capsicum/Cayenne is very high in iron, potassium and calcium.

*Catnip

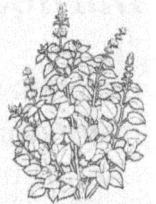

CATNIP is great for treating bronchitis. It treats colds, coughs and inflammation, it will expel gas and it treats insomnia. Catnip may be taken in capsules. If it is taken as a tea, use ¼ teaspoon of Catnip herb powder to one cup of boiling water. Catnip may be taken as often as you feel the need. For treating chronic bronchitis it may be taken two or three times a day, for two to seven days, or until desired results are reached. For some two or three times a week will be beneficial.

Herbs for your blood type: Catnip is neutral for people with O, B and AB. People with blood type A should avoid Catnip.

Contains: magnesium, sodium, iron, potassium, silicon, selenium, sulphur, and is rich in vitamins A, B complex, and C.

*Chamomile:

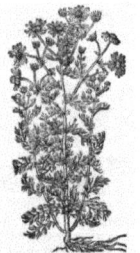

CHAMOMILE can be superb for treating bronchitis. It treats colds, fevers, flu, and nervousness. It treats poor circulation, cysts in the breast, and drug addiction. It stimulates the appetite. It may be taken in capsules. If it is taken as a tea, use ¼ teaspoon of Chamomile herb powder to one cup of boiling water. Chamomile may be taken as often as you feel the need. For treating chronic bronchitis it may be taken two or three times a day, for two to seven days, or until desired results are reached. For some two or three times a week can be beneficial.

Herbs for your blood type: Chamomile is highly beneficial for people with blood type A and AB. It is neutral for people with blood type O, and B.

Contains: potassium, calcium, iron, manganese, vitamin A, and zinc.

BRONCHITIS

*Chickweed

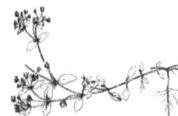

CHICKWEED is one of the best herbs for treating Bronchitis. It treats allergies, bronchial congestion, coughs, cancer, gout, and obesity. Chickweed will suppress the appetite. **Chickweed may elevate blood pressure for some people when taken excessively.** It may be taken in capsules. If it is taken as a tea, use ¼ teaspoon of Chickweed herb powder to one cup of boiling water. Chickweed may be taken as often as you feel the need. For chronic bronchitis it may be taken two or three times a day for two to five days, or until desired results are reached. For some two or three times a week will give desired results.

Herbs for your blood type: Chickweed is highly beneficial for people with blood type O. It is neutral for people with blood type A, B. and AB.

Contains: sodium, zinc, and B complex, and is high in iron, vitamin C, minerals, calcium, and copper.

Cinnamon

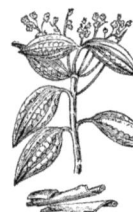

CINNAMON will help with the relief of bronchitis. It treats gas, nausea, cancer, rheumatism, vomiting, chest discomfort, and indigestion. Cinnamon may cause excessive menstrual flow. **Pregnant women should avoid Cinnamon during pregnancy. Men with prostate problems should also avoid Cinnamon. Diabetics should consult a health care provider before taking Cinnamon; some herbalists say it will increase insulin activity.** Cinnamon may be used as a spice in the kitchen. It may be taken in capsules. If it is taken as a tea, use ¼ teaspoon of Cinnamon herb powder to one cup of boiling water. Cinnamon may be taken as often as you feel the need. For chronic bronchitis it may be taken two or three times a day for two to five days, or until the desired results are reached. For some two or three times a week can be helpful.

Contains: calcium, chromium, copper, iodine, manganese, potassium, zinc, tannin, and vitamins A, B, and C.

BRONCHITIS

HERBS:

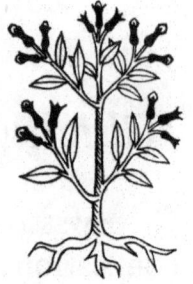

Cloves

CLOVES will assist with the treatment of bronchitis. It treats circulation, indigestion and vomiting. It treats nausea, bad breath, and dizziness. It may be taken in capsules. If Cloves is taken as a tea, use ¼ teaspoon of Cloves herb powder to one cup of boiling water. It is recommended that you purchase Cloves from an herb store; however Cloves purchased in the market will still be useful for treating a toothache.

Cloves may be taken as often as you feel the need. For treating bronchitis it may be taken two or three times a day, for two to seven days, or until desired results are reached. For some two or three times a week will give relief.

Contains: sodium, potassium, calcium, magnesium, phosphorus, vitamins A, B complex, and C.

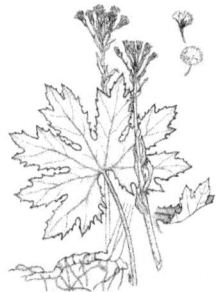

Coltsfoot

COLTSFOOT can be among the best herbs to use for bronchitis. It clears the lungs, treats asthma, coughs, inflammation, and pneumonia. Coltsfoot may be taken in capsules. If it is taken as a tea, use ¼ teaspoon of Coltsfoot herb powder to one cup of boiling water. Coltsfoot may be taken as often as you feel the need. For chronic bronchitis it may be taken once or twice a day, for two to five days, or until desired results are reached. For some two or three times a week will give relief.

Herbs for your blood type: Coltsfoot is neutral for people with blood type A. People with blood type O, B and AB should avoid this herb.

Contains: calcium, potassium, manganese, copper, zinc, vitamins P, B12, and B6, and a high amount of vitamins A and C.

BRONCHITIS

HERBS:

Comfrey

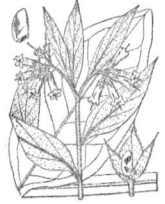

COMFREY can be helpful for treating bronchitis. It is soothing and helps with treating the digestive system. It treats anemia, asthma, bladder problems, and cancer sores. Comfrey may be taken in capsules. If it is taken as a tea, use ¼ teaspoon of Comfrey herb powder to one cup of boiling water. Comfrey may be taken as often as you feel the need. For bronchitis it may be taken two or three times a day, for two to seven days, or until desired results are reached. For some two or three times a week will be helpful.

Contains: vitamins A, C, iron, sulphur, copper, zinc and magnesium. Comfrey is very high in calcium, potassium and protein.

Couch Grass

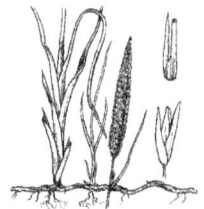

COUCH GRASS will help with the treatment of bronchitis. It treats urinary and bladder infections. It treats cystitis, enlarged prostate glands, female disorders and syphilis. It is very effective for treating bacteria and molds. Couch Grass may be taken in capsules. If it is taken as a tea, use ¼ teaspoon of Couch Grass herb powder to one cup of boiling water. Couch Grass may be taken as often as you feel the need. For treating bronchitis it may be taken once or twice a day, for two to seven days, or until desired results are reached. For some two or three times a week will give relief.

Contains: a high amount of silicon, vitamin A, C, and B complex. sodium, potassium, calcium, and magnesium.

BRONCHITIS

HERBS:

Damiana

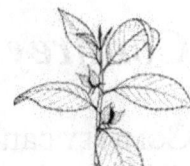

DAMIANA can be useful for treating bronchitis. It treats coughs, emphysema, and fatigue. It is an aphrodisiac that will enhance sexual desires in both men and women. It treats depression, exhaustion, prostate problems, and Parkinson's disease. It may be taken in capsules. If it is taken as a tea, use ¼ teaspoon of Damiana herb powder to one cup of boiling water. Damiana may be taken as often as you feel the need. For treating bronchitis it may be taken two or three times a day, for two to four days, or until desired results are reached. For some two or three times a week will give relief.

Contains: vitamins A and C, zinc, B complex, calcium, potassium, protein, selenium, and sodium.

Dandelion

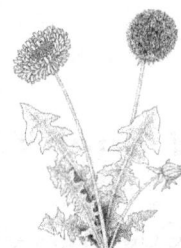

DANDELION will assist with treating bronchitis. It lowers cholesterol, treats breast cancer, and female organs. It treats liver problems and senility. Dandelion will increase urine flow. **Dandelion may elevate blood pressure for some people when taken excessively.** It is a bitter herb and it may be taken in capsules. If it is taken as a tea, use ¼ teaspoon of Dandelion herb powder to one cup of boiling water. Dandelion may be taken as often as you feel the need. For treating bronchitis it may be taken two or three times a day, for two to four days, or until desired results are reached. For some, two or three times a week will give relief.

Herbs for your blood type: Dandelion is highly beneficial for people with blood type O. It is neutral for people with blood type A, B, and AB.

Contains: calcium, vitamin A, B, C, and E, sodium, potassium, iron, nickel, tin copper magnesium, manganese, sulphur, and zinc.

BRONCHITIS

HERBS:

Dong Quai

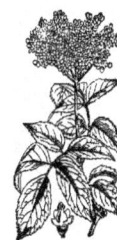

DONG QUAI can be helpful for treating bronchitis. It treats nervousness, poor circulation, and cancer. It purifies the blood and treats female problems. Dong Quai may be taken in capsules. If it is taken as a tea, use ¼ teaspoon of Dong Quai herb powder to one cup of boiling water. Dong Quai may be taken as often as you feel the need. For treating bronchitis it may be taken two or three times a day until the desired results are reached. For some, two or three times a week will give relief.

Herbs for your blood type: Dong Quai is neutral for people with blood type O, A, B and AB.

Contains: a high amount of iron, it also has vitamins A, B12, and E.

*Elder Flower

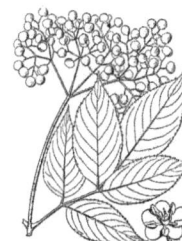

ELDER FLOWER is excellent for treating bronchitis. It clears the lungs, treats asthma, pneumonia, fevers and cancer. Elder Flower may be taken in capsules. If it is taken as a tea, use ¼ teaspoon of Elder Flower herb powder to one cup of boiling water. Elder Flower may be taken as often as you feel the need. For treating bronchitis it may be taken two or three times a day, for two to five days, or until desired results are reached. For some, two or three times a week will give relief.

Herbs for your blood type: Elder Flower is neutral for people with blood type O, A, B and AB.

Contains: vitamins A and C.

BRONCHITIS

HERBS:

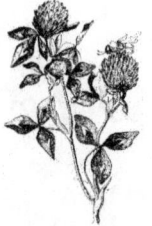

*Elecampane

ELECAMPANE is excellent for treating chronic bronchitis. It treats asthma, coughs, respiratory problems, and emphysema. It will increase the appetite; it will lower sugar levels in the blood. Elecampane is best used in combination with other herbs. It may be taken in capsules. If it is taken as a tea, use ¼ teaspoon of Elecampane herb powder to one cup of boiling water. Elecampane may be taken as often as you feel the need. For treating chronic bronchitis it may be taken once or twice a day, for two to seven days, or until the desired results are reached. For some, two or three times a week will give relief.

Contains: sodium, calcium, and potassium.

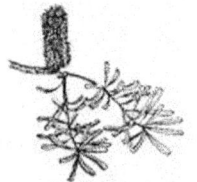

*Eucalyptus

EUCALYPTUS may be used as a vapor for treating bronchitis. For vapor use one teaspoon of Eucalyptus oil as a steamer.

BRONCHITIS

Fennel

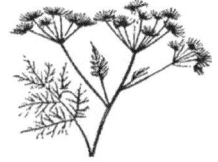

FENNEL will help with treating bronchitis. It treats the digestive system, emphysema, coughs and food poisoning. **Fennel may increase the blood pressure for some people if it is taken excessively.** Fennel may be taken in capsules. If it is taken as a tea, use ¼ teaspoon of Fennel herb powder to one cup of boiling water. Fennel may be taken as often as you feel the need. For treating bronchitis it may be taken once or twice a day, for two to five days, or until the desired results are reached. For some, two or three times a week will give relief.

Contains: sodium, potassium, and sulphur, and is high in vitamin A.

*Fenugreek

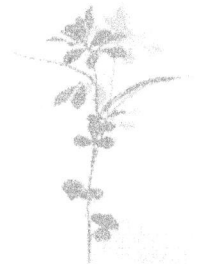

FENUGREEK is a must-have for treating bronchitis. It treats allergies, emphysema, lung infections, and mucus membranes. Fenugreek should not be used by women that wish to get pregnant, it will impede the progress. It may be taken in capsules. If it is taken as a tea, use ¼ teaspoon of Fenugreek herb powder to one cup of boiling water. Fenugreek may be taken as often as you feel the need. For treating chronic bronchitis it may be taken two or three times a day, for two to five days, or until desired results are reached. For some, two or three times a week will give relief.

Herbs for your blood type: Fenugreek is highly beneficial for people with blood type O, and A. People with blood type B, and AB should not use this herb.

Contains: B1, B2, iron, choline, and is rich in vitamins A and D.

BRONCHITIS

HERBS:

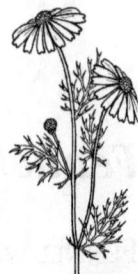

Feverfew

FEVERFEW will help with the treatment of bronchitis. It treats allergies, colds, digestive problems, and hay fever. It treats fevers, migraine headaches and painful arthritis. Feverfew may be taken in capsules. If it is taken as a tea, use ¼ teaspoon of Fever Few herb powder to one cup of boiling water. Feverfew may be taken as often as you feel the need. For treating bronchitis it may be taken two or three times a day, for two to five days, or until desired results are reached. For some, two or three times a week will give relief.

Contains: sodium, and Vitamin A, C, and zinc, and a high amount of iron, niacin, potassium manganese, and phosphorus.

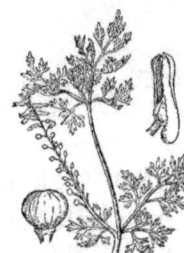

Fumitory

FUMITORY will assist with the treatment of bronchitis. It treats constipation, hemorrhoids, liver problems, rheumatism, and stomach disorders. Fumitory is a diuretic and it lowers blood pressure. Use Fumitory sparingly or it will cause stomach cramps. Fumitory may be taken in capsules. If it is taken as a tea, use 1/8th teaspoon of Fumitory herb powder, or less to one cup of boiling water. Fumitory may be taken as often as you feel the need. For treating bronchitis it may be taken once a day, for one to two days, or until desired results are reached.

Content: vitamin information unknown.

BRONCHITIS

HERBS:

*Garlic

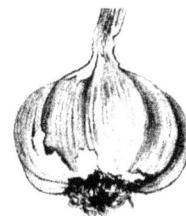

GARLIC is excellent for treating chronic bronchitis. It treats asthma, digestive disorders, lungs, prostate problems and ear infections. Garlic may elevate blood pressure for some people when taken excessively. Garlic may be taken in capsules. If it is taken as a tea, use ¼ teaspoon of Garlic herb powder to one cup of boiling water. Garlic may be taken as often as you feel the need. For treating chronic bronchitis it may be taken two or three times a day, for two to seven days, or until the desired results are reached. For some, two or three times a week will give relief. Herbs for your blood type: Garlic is highly beneficial for people with blood type A and AB. It is neutral for people with blood type O and B.

Contains: sodium, sulphur, calcium, copper, vitamin B1, iron, and is high in potassium, zinc selenium, vitamins A and C.

Ginseng/Panax

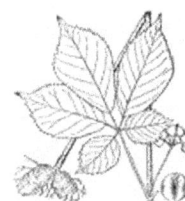

GINSENG/PANAX will help to treat bronchitis. It stimulates the lungs, offers radiation protection, and stimulates the appetite. Ginseng/Panax will increase energy, sexual endurance, and it helps to bring hormones into balance. Ginseng/Panax increases male hormones and helps with impotency. Long-term use is not recommended for women, it will produce testosterone. This herb will benefit men on long term just great! Ginseng/Panax is best prepared in glass cookware, as metal pots will reduce the strength. It may be taken in capsules. If it is taken as a tea, use ¼ teaspoon of Ginseng/Panax herb powder to one cup of boiling water. Ginseng/Panax may be taken as often as you feel the need. For treating bronchitis it may be taken once or twice a day, for two to five days, or until the desired results are reached. For some, two or three times a week will give relief.

Herbs for your blood type: Ginseng is highly beneficial for Blood types O, A, B, and AB.

Contains: vitamins A, B12, E, iron, calcium, magnesium, sodium, sulphur, niacin, potassium, silicon, manganese, and phosphorus.

BRONCHITIS

*Golden Seal

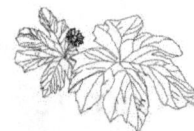

GOLDEN SEAL works great for treating chronic bronchitis. It treats, colds coughs, infections and contagious diseases. It will reduce sugar in the blood when it is used in combination with the licorice herb. Myrrh should be used with this herb if you suffer low blood sugar. Pregnant women should not use Golden Seal during pregnancy. **Golden Seal may elevate the blood pressure for some people when taken excessively.** Golden Seal is a bitter herb. It may be taken in capsules. If it is taken as a tea, use ¼ teaspoon of Golden Seal herb powder to one cup of boiling water. Golden Seal may be taken as often as you feel the need. For treating bronchitis it may be taken once or twice a day, for two to five days, or until desired results are reached. For some, two or three times a week will give relief.

Herbs for your blood type: Golden Seal is neutral for people with blood type A, B and AB. People with blood type O should avoid this herb.

Contains: calcium, potassium, iron, zinc, sodium, and vitamins A, C, B complex, and E.

*Gumweed

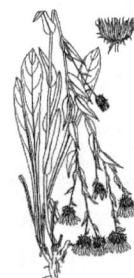

GUMWEED can be superb to use for treating chronic bronchitis. It treats asthma, bladder infections, psoriasis and bronchial irritation. Gumweed should be used in combination with other herbs. Use a very small amount of Gumweed at once. Use less than 1/8th teaspoon of Gumweed. This herb is not recommended for people with heart problems. If it is taken as a tea use a small pinch to one cup of boiling water. Gumweed may be taken once a day for not more than two days a week, until desired results are reached.

Contains: lead, tin, zinc, and some arsenic.

CANCER

Agrimony

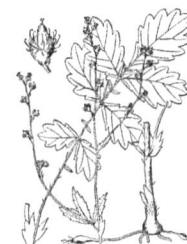

AGRIMONY can be especially useful for treating cancer. It treats cancer of the kidneys, liver, colon, and stomach. The throat will also receive benefits. Agrimony is a tonic that is high in nutrients. It may be taken in capsules. If it is taken as a tea, use ¼ teaspoon of Agrimony herb powder to one cup of boiling water. Agrimony may be taken as often as you feel the need. For treating cancer it may be taken once or twice a day, for two to ten days, or until desired results are reached. For some, two or three times a week will be beneficial.

Contains: iron, niacin, vitamin K, and B3.

*Alfafa

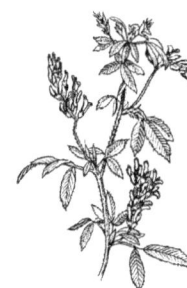

ALFALFA can be great for helping to preventing colon cancer. It neutralizes cancer in the system when taken regularly. Alfalfa wards off infections and stimulates the pituitary gland. It treats urinary and bowel problems, and acidity. It may be taken in capsules. If it is taken as a tea, use ¼ teaspoon of Alfalfa herb powder to one cup of boiling water. Alfalfa may be taken as often as you feel the need. For treating cancer it may be taken once or twice a day, for three to five days, or until the desired results are reached. For some, two or three times a week will be beneficial.

Herbs for your blood type: Alfalfa is highly beneficial for people with blood type A. It is neutral for people with blood type B and AB. People with blood type O should avoid this herb it will cause excessive blood thinning for them.

CANCER

HERBS:

Contains: vitamins A, B complex, D, E, and K, iron, potassium, magnesium, protein, sodium, sulfur, phosphorus, and is very high in calcium, chlorophyll, and vitamin B12.

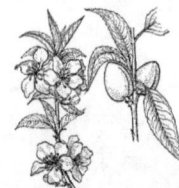

Almond

ALMOND can be helpful for treating cancer. It treats cancer caused from tension. This is a bitter herb and it may be taken in capsules. If it is taken as a tea, use ¼ teaspoon of Almond herb powder to one cup of boiling water. Almond may be taken as often as you feel the need. For treating cancer it may be taken once or twice a day for two, to seven days, or until the desired results are reached. For some, two or three times a week will be beneficial.

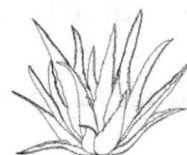

Aloe

ALOE can be extremely useful for helping to treat cancer. It will boost the immune system, help to remove toxins from the body, and stimulate normal growth of living cells. It can be helpful for any type of damage caused from radiation or chemotherapy. Aloe Vera is a bitter herb, and it may be taken in capsules. If it is taken as a tea, use ¼ teaspoon of Aloe herb powder to one cup of boiling water. Or, wash whole Aloe Vera leaves in warm water; remove the side thorns, and place the leaves in a juicer, do not add sugar. Juice four to six ounces and drink it immediately. Aloe Vera may be taken as often as you feel the need. For treating cancer it may be taken once or twice a day, for three to seven days, or until the desired results are reached. For some, two or three times a week will be beneficial.

Herbs for your blood type: Aloe is highly beneficial for people with blood type A. People with blood type O, B and AB should avoid the herb.

Contains: potassium, sodium, manganese, iron, and zinc.

CANCER

Astragalus

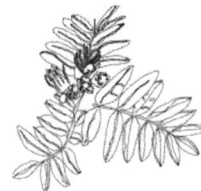

ASTRAGALUS can be helpful with treating cancer; it helps when cancer is being treated with chemotherapy. It treats chronic fatigue, heals damaged tissues, treats the uterus, and eliminates toxins from the system. Astragalus increases white T-cells, and stimulates the immune system. Urination increases while taking Astragalus, it is a diuretic. It may be taken in capsules. If it is taken as a tea, use ¼ teaspoons of Astragalus herb powder to one cup of boiling water. Astragalus may be taken as often as you feel the need. For cancer it may be taken two or three times a day for two to seven days, or until the desired results are reached. For some, two or three times a week will be beneficial.

Contains: choline, betaine, and gluconic acid.

Barberry

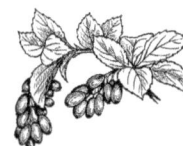

BARBERRY can be very helpful for treating cancer; it purifies the blood, cleans the liver, treats infections in the body, it stimulates the appetite. It dilates blood vessels, which makes it good for high blood pressure. **Do not take Barberry excessively at once; it may cause depression.** Barberry may be taken in capsules, if it is taken as a tea; use 1/8th teaspoon or less of Barberry herb powder to one cup of boiling water. Barberry may be taken as often as you feel the need. For treating cancer it may be taken once a day, for two to five days, or until the desired results are reached. For some, two or three times a week will be beneficial for two to four weeks.

Contains: iron, manganese, phosphorus, and vitamin C.

CANCER

HERBS:

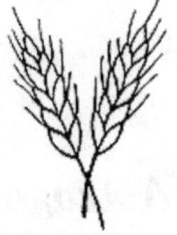

*Barley Juice Powder

BARLEY JUICE POWDER is excellent for treating cancer; it will boost the immune system as it cleans the blood cells. It helps to remove metals, mercury, and lead from the blood. It helps to lower cholesterol. Barley Juice Powder may be taken in capsules. If it is taken as a tea, use ¼ teaspoon of Barley Juice herb powder to one cup of boiling water. Or, you may juice the fresh leaves of barley and drink it immediately. Barley Juice Powder may be taken as often as you feel the need. For treating cancer it may be taken once or twice a day, for three to seven days, or until the desired results are reached. For some, two or three times a week will be beneficial until desired results are reached.

Contains: vitamins B1, B12, C, potassium and is high in iron and calcium.

Bee Pollen

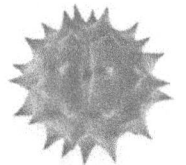

BEE POLLEN will help to treat cancer; it will stimulate the appetite, it treats fatigue, builds energy, and it treats exhaustion. It will assist with treating prostate disorders. Bee Pollen will boost the immune system during radiation treatments. Bee Pollen treats early stages of multiple sclerosis. It is best to begin taking small amounts of this herb in the beginning and increase it as your system adjusts to it. It rejuvenates the whole body as it builds the blood. It may be taken in capsules. If it is taken as a tea, use ¼ teaspoon of Bee Pollen herb powder to one cup of boiling water. Bee Pollen may be taken as often as you feel the need. For treating cancer it may be taken once or twice a day, for three to seven days, or until desired results are reached. For some, two or three times a week can be helpful.

Contains: vitamin C, B complex, enzymes, iron, magnesium, manganese, potassium, sodium, and amino acids.

CANCER

Birch

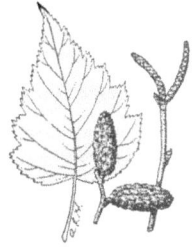

BIRCH will help with treating cancer; it is a blood cleanser, and it offers a sedative effect, it treats vomiting and it assists with treating the pain. Birch may be taken in capsules. If it is taken as a tea, use ¼ teaspoon of Birch herb powder to one cup of boiling water. Birch may be taken as often as you feel the need. For treating cancer it may be taken two or three times a day, for three to five days, or until desired results are reached. For some, two or three times a week will be beneficial.

Contains: copper, sodium, calcium, iron, magnesium, potassium, silicon, and vitamins A, B1, B2, C, and E.

Black Cohosh

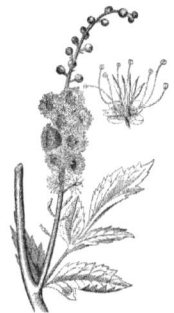

BLACK COHOSH will help with treating cancer; it cleanses and treats cancer in the lymphatic system. It cleans the blood, it lowers the heart rate slightly, and increases the pulse rate, it reduces hot flashes and it is a sedative. **Black Cohosh will induce labor when pregnant. Black Cohosh should be used in small amounts or it can cause a headache.** Black Cohosh may be taken in capsules. If it is taken as a tea, use 1/8th teaspoon or less, of Black Cohosh herb powder to one cup of boiling water. Black Cohosh may be taken as often as you feel the need. For treating cancer it may be taken once or twice a day, for three to five days, or until the desired results are reached. For some, two or three times a week will be beneficial.

Contains: calcium, potassium, iron, magnesium, manganese, niacin, phosphorus, selenium, silicon, sodium, sulphur, zinc vitamins A, B1, B2, C, K, and F.

CANCER

HERBS:

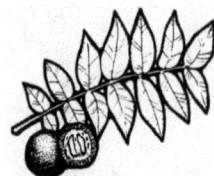

Black Walnut

BLACK WALNUT will help with the treatment of cancer; it treats diseased blood, herpes, and it kills parasites in the blood. It has high organic iodine content and it helps to balance sugar levels. Black Walnut may be taken in capsules. If it is taken as a tea, use ¼ teaspoon of Black Walnut herb powder to one cup of boiling water. Black Walnut may be taken as often as you feel the need. For treating cancer it may be taken two or three times a day for three to seven days, or until the desired results are reached. For some, once or twice a week will be beneficial.

Contains: magnesium, potassium, iron, calcium, and vitamin B15.

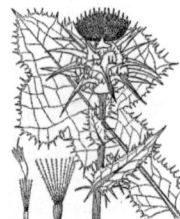

*Blessed Thistle

BLESSED THISTLE is also known as Holy Thistle. It treats cancer in the organs. It purifies the blood and increases oxygen to the brain, helps with liver disorders, increases the appetite, improves circulation and strengthens the heart. It may be taken in capsules. If it is taken as a tea, use ¼ teaspoon of Blessed Thistle herb powder to one cup of boiling water. Blessed Thistle may be taken as often as you feel the need. For treating cancer it may be taken once or twice a day, for three to seven days, or until the desired results are reached. For some, two or three times a week will be beneficial.

Contains: B complex, calcium, iron, manganese and potassium.

CANCER

HERBS:

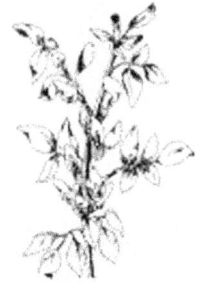

Broad Bean

BROAD BEAN can be effective with treating cancer; it cleans the lymphatic system. It increases energy, treats herpes, and Parkinson's disease. Broad Bean is a diuretic and may be taken in capsules. If it is taken as a tea, use ¼ teaspoon of Broad Bean herb powder to one cup of boiling water. Broad Bean may be taken as often as you feel the need. For treating cancer it may be taken once or twice a day, for three to five days, or until the desired results are reached. For some, two or three times a week will be beneficial.

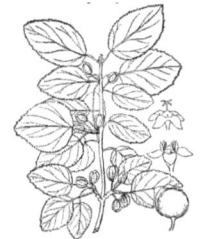

*Buckthorn

BUCKTHORN is excellent for treating cancer; it cleans the blood and removes lead from the system. Buckthorn also works as a laxative. **Buckthorn may cause stomach cramping when taken excessively at once.** It may be taken in capsules. If it is taken as a tea, use ¼ teaspoon of Buckthorn herb powder to one cup of boiling water. Buckthorn may be taken as often as you feel the need. For treating cancer it may be taken once or twice a day, for three to five days, or until the desired results are reached. For some, two or three times a week will be beneficial.

Contains vitamin C.

CANCER

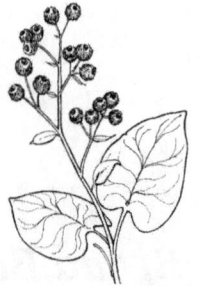

*Burdock

BURDOCK can be great for treating cancer; it purifies the blood, and cleans the lymphatic system. Burdock increases urine flow. Burdock may cause vomiting when taken excessively at once. Burdock may be taken in capsules. If it is taken as a tea, use ¼ teaspoon of Burdock herb powder, to one cup of boiling water. Burdock may be taken as often as you feel the need. For treating cancer it may be taken once or twice a day, for three to five days, or until the desired results are reached. For some, two or three times a week will be beneficial.

Herbs for your blood type: Burdock is highly beneficial for people with blood type A and AB. It is neutral for people with blood type B. People with blood type O should avoid this herb it will cause excessive blood thinning and excessive bleeding for them.

Contains: vitamins A, B complex, C, E, iron, zinc, and sulphur.

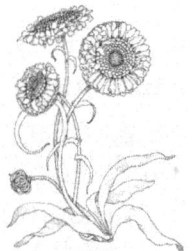

Calendula

CALENDULA will helpful with the treatment of cancer; it cleanses and purifies the blood. It treats internal and external bleeding, especially if there are sores. It may be taken in capsules, if it is taken as a tea use 1/8th teaspoon of Calendula herb powder to one cup of boiling water. Calendula may be taken as often as you feel the need. For treating cancer it may be taken once a day, for two to five days, or until the desired results are reached. For some, two or three times a week can be helpful.

Content: vitamin information unknown.

CANCER

HERBS:

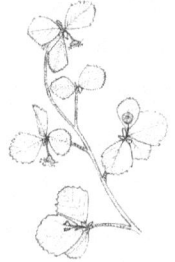

*Chaparral

CHAPARRAL dissolves cancer cells; it treats tumors, leukemia, cleans the lymphatic system and purifies the blood. Chaparral may be taken in capsules. If it is taken as a tea, use ¼ teaspoon of Chaparral herb powder to one cup of boiling water. Chaparral may be taken as often as you feel the need. For treating cancer it may be taken once or twice a day, for two to seven days, or until the desired results are reached. For some, two or three times a week will be beneficial.

Contains: sodium, potassium, aluminum, barium, chlorine, protein, silicon, and sulphur.

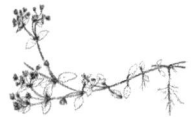

*Chickweed

CHICKWEED is excellent for treating cancer; it treats cancerous tumors. It dissolves plaque in the blood and other fatty substances. Chickweed will suppress the appetite. It may be taken in capsules. If it is taken as a tea, use ¼ teaspoon of Chickweed herb powder to one cup of boiling water. Chickweed may be taken as often as you feel the need. For treating cancer it may be taken once or twice a day, for three to seven days, or until the desired results are reached. For some, two or three times a week will be beneficial.

Herbs for your blood type: Chickweed is highly beneficial for people with blood type O. It is neutral for people with blood type A, B, and AB.

Contains: sodium zinc and B complex and is high in iron, vitamin C, minerals, calcium, and copper.

CANCER

HERBS:

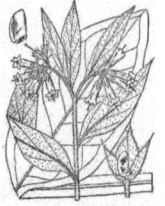

Comfrey

COMFREY will assist with treating cancer; it stimulates new cell growth for rapid cancer healing. It is an excellent blood cleanser. It treats emphysema, pneumonia, and tuberculosis. It treats gangrene sores, infections and bloody urine. It may be taken in capsules. If it is taken as a tea, use ¼ teaspoon of Comfrey herb powder to one cup of boiling water. Comfrey may be taken as often as you feel the need. For treating cancer it may be taken once or twice a day, for five to seven days, or until the desired results are reached. For some, two or three times a week will be beneficial.

Contains: vitamins A, C, iron, sulphur, copper, zinc and magnesium. Comfrey is very high in calcium, potassium and protein.

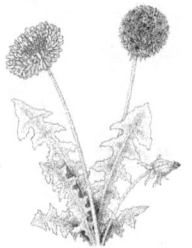

Dandelion

DANDELION will be helpful with treating breast cancer; it treats tumors in the breast and it can be used as a poultice on the breast. It treats fatigue, water retention, uric acid, acne, and arthritis. **Dandelion may elevate blood pressure for some people when taken excessively.** Dandelion may be taken in capsules. If it is taken as a tea, use ¼ teaspoon of Dandelion herb powder to one cup of boiling water. Dandelion may be taken as often as you feel the need. For treating cancer it may be taken once or twice a day, for two to seven days, or until the desired results are reached. For some, three or four times a week will be helpful.

Herbs for your blood type: Dandelion is highly beneficial for people with blood type O. It is neutral for people with blood type A, B, and AB.

Contains: calcium, vitamin A, B, C, E, sodium, potassium, iron, nickel, tin copper magnesium, manganese, sulphur, and zinc.

CANCER

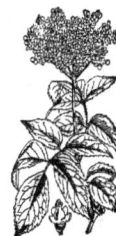

Dong Quai

DONG QUAI can assist with treating cancer; it cleans the lymphatic system. Dong Quai, Chaparral and Red Clover makes a good combination for treating cancer. Dong Quai will strengthen the circulation and purify the blood. Dong Quai may be taken in capsules. If it is taken as a tea, use ¼ teaspoon of Dong Quai herb powder to one cup of boiling water. Dong Quai may be taken as often as you feel the need. For treating cancer it may be taken once or twice a day, for two to five days, or until the desired results are reached. For some, two or three times a week will be beneficial.

Herbs for your blood type: Dong Quai is neutral for people with blood type O, A, B and AB."

Contains: vitamins A, B12 and E magnesium, manganese, nicotinic acid, phosphorus, potassium, silicon, sodium, B complex, C, E, and zinc, and is very high in iron

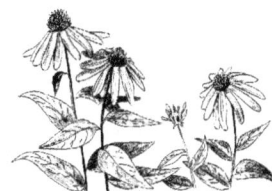

*Echinacea

ECHINACEA can be excellent for treating cancer; it cleans the lymphatic system, purifies the blood, stimulates and supports the immune system. It expels toxins and poisons from the system and prevents infections. Echinacea increases white blood cells. It may be taken in capsules. If it is taken as a tea, use ¼ teaspoon of Echinacea herb powder to one cup of boiling water. Echinacea may be taken as often as you feel the need. For treating cancer it may be taken once or twice a day, for two to five days, or until the desired results are reached. For some, two or three times a week will be beneficial.

Herbs for your blood type: Echinacea is highly beneficial for people with blood type A and AB. It is neutral for people with blood type B. People with blood type O should avoid this herb; it will cause excessive blood thinning for them"

Contains: vitamins A, C, E, iron, iodine, copper, sulphur, and potassium.

CANCER

HERBS:

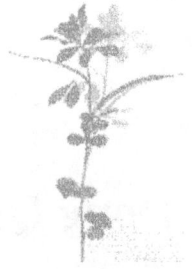

Fenugreek

FENUGREEK will assist with the treatment of cancer; it treats the lymphatic system, expels toxins from the body, and dissolves cholesterol. Fenugreek should not be used by women who which to get pregnant, it will impede the progress. It may be taken in capsules. If it is taken as a tea, use ¼ teaspoon of Fenugreek herb powder to one cup of boiling water. Fenugreek may be taken as often as you feel the need. For treating cancer it may be taken once or twice a day, for two to seven days, or until the desired results are reached. For some, two or three times a week will be beneficial.

Herbs for your blood type: Fenugreek is highly beneficial for people with blood type O, and A. People with blood type B, and AB should not use this herb.

Contains: B1, B2, iron and choline, and is very rich in vitamins A and D.

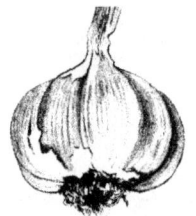

*Garlic

GARLIC can be excellent for treating cancer; it builds the immune system; it purifies the blood, treats poor circulation and treats ear infections. **Garlic may elevate blood pressure for some people when taken excessively.** It may be taken in capsules. If it is taken as a tea, use ¼ teaspoon of Garlic herb powder to one cup of boiling water. Garlic may be taken as often as you feel the need. For treating cancer it may be taken once or twice a day, for two to ten days, or until the desired results are reached. For some, two or three times a week will be beneficial.

Herbs for your blood type: Garlic is highly beneficial for people with blood type A and AB. It is neutral for people with blood type O and B.

Contains: sodium, sulphur, calcium, copper, vitamin B1, iron and is high in potassium, zinc selenium, vitamins A and C.

SYLVIA GILL

CANCER

HERBS:

Ginkgo

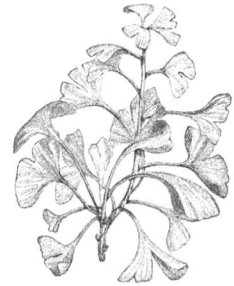

GINKGO will help with the treatment of cancer; it destroys free radicals in the system and improves the blood and other circulatory problems. Ginkgo may be taken in capsules. If it is taken as a tea, use ¼ teaspoon of Ginkgo to one cup of boiling water. Ginkgo may be taken as often as you feel the need. For treating cancer it may be taken once or twice a day, for two to five days, or until the desired results are reached. For some, two or three times a week will be beneficial.

Contains bioflavonoids.

Ginseng/Siberian

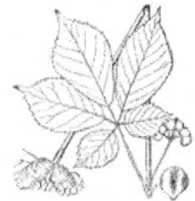

GINSENG/SIBERIAN can be helpful with treating cancer; it will be especially helpful when radiation is being used, it fights against fatigue, stimulates the appetite, and increases endurance. Ginseng/Siberian may be taken in capsules. If it is taken as a tea, use ¼ teaspoon of Ginseng Siberian herb powder to one cup of boiling water. Ginseng/Siberian may be taken as often as you feel the need. For treating cancer it may be taken once or twice a day, for two to seven days, or until the desired results are reached. For some, two or three times a week will be beneficial.

   Ginseng is highly beneficial for people with blood type A, B and AB. It is neutral for people with blood type O.

Contains: B12, sulphur, calcium, iron, sodium, and potassium.

135

CANCER

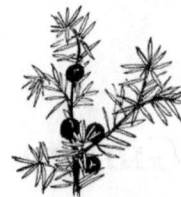

Juniper

JUNIPER can assist with treating cancer; if this herb is taken early before major damage has been done to the lymphatic system it will tone and heal the pancreas. It increases urine flow while it purifies the blood. Do not take Juniper if you suffer kidney disease, because it may over stimulate the kidneys and adrenals. Juniper may be taken in capsules, if it is taken as a tea, add ¼ teaspoon of Juniper to one cup of boiling water. Juniper may be taken as often as you feel the need. For treating cancer it may be taken once or twice a day, for two to seven days, or until the desired results are reached. For some, two or three times a week will be beneficial.

Contains: sulphur, copper, and a small amount of aluminum, and has a high amount of vitamin C.

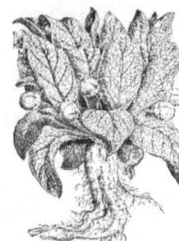

*Mandrake

MANDRAKE is great for dissolving cancerous tumors. This herb must be used in very small doses in combination with other herbs; it will gripe the stomach when used in large amounts: it is a laxative. **Do not use this herb during pregnancy.** It may be taken in capsules. When it is taken as a tea, use 1/8th teaspoon or less of Mandrake herb powder to two cups of boiling water. Mandrake may be taken as often as you feel the need. For treating cancer it may be taken once or twice a day, for two to five days, or until the desired results are reached. For some, once or twice a week will be beneficial.

Contents: vitamin information unknown.

CANCER

*Mullein

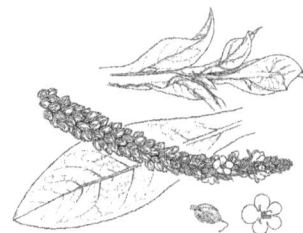

MULLEIN can be an excellent choice for treating cancer; it treats pain, and congestion in the lymphatic system, it treats swollen glands. Mullen offers treatment to lung disease. It may be taken in capsules. If it is taken as a tea, use ¼ teaspoon of Mullein herb powder to one cup of boiling water. Mullein may be taken as often as you feel the need. For treating cancer it may be taken once or twice a day, for two to seven days, or until the desired results are reached. For some, two or three times a week will be beneficial.

Herbs for your blood type: Mullein is neutral for people with blood type O and A. People with Blood type B and AB should avoid this herb."

Contains: magnesium, potassium and sulphur, and is very high in iron.

*Pau D'Arco

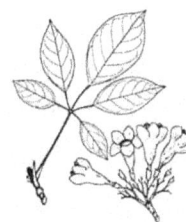

PAU D'ARCO will eases the pain of cancer; it can be very beneficial for treating Hodgkin's disease, and Leukemia. Pau D'Arco will boost the immune system and remove toxins and tumors. Pau D'Arco may be taken in capsules. If it is taken as a tea, use ¼ teaspoon of Pau D'Arco herb powder to one cup of boiling water. Pau D'Arco may be taken as often as you feel the need. For treating cancer it may be taken once or twice a day, for two to five days, or until the desired results are reached. For some, two or three times a week will be beneficial.

Contains: potassium, sodium, magnesium, manganese, selenium, and zinc. Vitamins A, B complex, and C, and is very high in iron.

CANCER

HERBS:

*Peach Bark

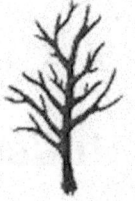

PEACH BARK is excellent for the treatment of cancer; it treats nausea and vomiting; it reduces tumors and cleans the blood. It helps to relieve gas and colic. Pregnant women should not take Peach Bark it can cause miscarriage. Peach Bark may be taken in capsules. If it is taken as a tea, use ½ teaspoon of Peach Bark herb powder to one cup of boiling water. Peach Bark may be taken as often as you feel the need. For treating cancer it may be taken once a day, for two to five days, or until the desired results are reached. For some, once or twice a week will be beneficial.

Content: vitamin information unknown

*Periwinkle

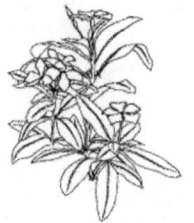

PERIWINKLE is an excellent herb for treating cancer; it treats Hodgkin's disease, leukemia and carries oxygen to the brain. Periwinkle acts as a sedative. Periwinkle may be taken in capsules. If it is taken as a tea, use ¼ teaspoon of Periwinkle herb powder to one cup of boiling water. Periwinkle may be taken as often as you feel the need. For treating cancer it may be taken once or twice a day until the desired results are reached. For some, two or three times a week will be beneficial.

Content: vitamin information unknown.

CANCER

HERBS:

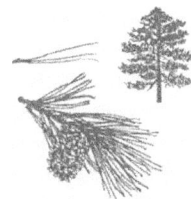

*Pine Tree Bark

PINE TREE BARK is among the best herbs for treating cancer. It treats the lymphatic system, rebuilds tissues in the body, improves circulation of the blood, and increases memory. Pine Tree Bark makes many corrections within the body. It may be taken in capsules. If it is taken as a tea, use ¼ teaspoon of Pine Tree Bark herb powder to one cup of boiling water. Pine Tree Bark may be taken as often as you feel the need. For treating cancer it may be taken once or twice a day, for two to five days, or until desired results is reached.. For some, once or twice a week can be very beneficial.

Content: vitamin information unknown.

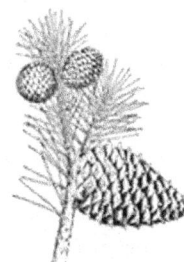

Prickly Ash

PRICKLY ASH can help to treat cancer; it helps to treat peripheral lymphatic cancer; it purifies the blood and improves poor circulation. It increases the flow of saliva in the mouth. Prickly Ash will increase circulation to the legs. It treats a wide variety of conditions. It warms cold hands, cold feet, and cold legs. It may cause some people to become more sensitive to sunlight and burn more easily. It helps to treat yeast growth and gonorrhea. Prickly Ash can be taken in capsules. If it is taken as a tea, use ¼ teaspoon of prickly ash herb powder to one cup of boiling water. Prickly Ash may be taken as often as you feel the need. For treating cancer it may be taken once or twice a day, for two to five days, or until desired results are reached. For some, two or three times a week will be beneficial.

Contains tannins.

CANCER

HERBS:

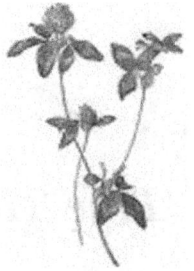

*Red Clover

RED CLOVER treats cancer anywhere in the body; it increases energy, cleans and purifies the blood. Red Clover may be taken in capsules. If it is taken as a tea, use ¼ teaspoon of Red Clover herb powder to one cup of boiling water. Red Clover may be taken as often as you feel the need. For treating cancer it may be taken once or twice a day for two to five days at a time. For some, once or twice a week can be beneficial.

Contains: vitamins A, B complex, calcium, sodium, nickel, manganese, tin, and is high in iron, and calcium.

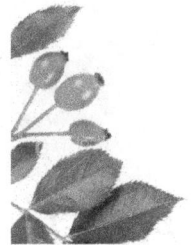

*Rose Hips

ROSE HIPS is an excellent choice for the prevention of cancer. It purifies the blood, increases energy and treats infections. For people that are allergic to citrus, Rose Hips is an excellent alternative to vitamin C. Rose Hips may be taken in capsules. If it is taken as a tea, use ¼ teaspoon of Rose Hips herb powder to one cup of boiling water. Rose Hips may be taken as often as you feel the need. For cancer prevention/treatment it may be taken once or twice a day, for two to seven days, or until the desired results are reached. For some, two or three times a week can be beneficial.

Contains: vitamins A, B complex, and E, sodium, potassium, iron, niacin and sulphur, and a higher content of vitamin C than citrus.

CANCER

Suma

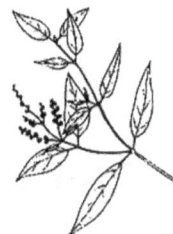

SUMA can be very beneficial for treating cancer; it treats Hodgkin's disease and leukemia. It increases new cell growth and prevents the release of free radicals. It boosts the immune system and increases vitality. Suma enhances sexual function for both men and women. It may be taken in capsules. If it is taken as a tea, use ¼ teaspoon of Suma herb powder to one cup of boiling water. Suma may be taken as often as you feel the need. For treating cancer it may be taken once or twice a day, for two to five days, or until the desired results are reached. For some, two or three times a week will be beneficial for three to four weeks.

Contains: iron, magnesium, vitamin B complex, minerals, and amino acids.

Violet

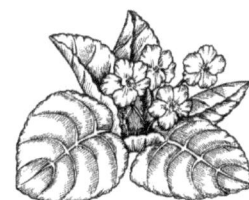

VIOLET is a good choice to use as a poultice for skin cancer. When used as a poultice it works well for the breast and lungs. It is excellent after surgery to prevent tumors from returning. Violet may be taken in capsules, if it is taken as a tea, use ¼ teaspoon of Violet herb powder to one cup of boiling water. Violet may be taken as often as you feel the need. For treating cancer it may be taken once or twice a day, for two to seven days, or until the desired results are reached. For some, two or three times a week will be beneficial for three to four weeks.

Contains: vitamins A and C.

CANCER

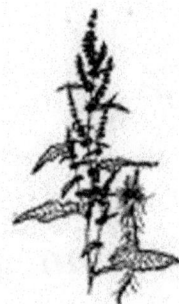

*Yellow Dock

YELLOW DOCK is excellent for treating cancer; it treats and cleans the lymphatic system. It builds the immune system, cleans and purifies the blood. This is one of the best blood builders known. Yellow Dock may be taken in capsules. If it is taken as a tea, use ¼ teaspoon of Yellow Dock herb powder to one cup of boiling water. Yellow Dock may be taken as often as you feel the need. For treating cancer it may be taken once or twice a day, for two to seven days, or until the desired results are reached. For some, two or three times a week will be beneficial for three to four weeks.

Yellow Dock is neutral for people with blood type B and AB. People with blood type O, and A should avoid this herb.

Contains: vitamins A and C, nickel, and is very high in iron.

CIRCULATION

Bayberry

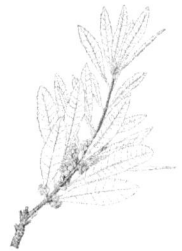

BAYBERRY helps to improve circulation. It is a tonic that stimulates and strengthens the entire body. Bayberry offers vitality to the body. It may be taken in capsules. If it is taken as a tea, use ¼ teaspoon of Bayberry herb powder to one cup of boiling water. Bayberry may be taken as often as you feel the need. For poor circulation it may be taken two or three times a day for two to five days, or until desired results are reached. For some, once or twice a week will be helpful for two to three weeks or until desired results are reached.

Contains: calcium, sodium, magnesium, manganese, niacin, potassium, silicon, phosphorus, zinc, vitamins B1, B2, and C.

*Blessed Thistle

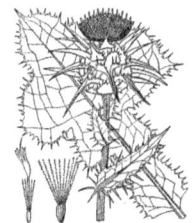

BLESSED THISTLE is also known as Holy; increases blood circulation; it brings oxygen to the brain and throughout the system. Blessed Thistle treats cancer, calcium deposits, and strengthens the heart. It may be taken in capsules. If it is taken as a tea, use ¼ teaspoon of Blessed Thistle herb powder to one cup of boiling water. Blessed Thistle may be taken as often as you feel the need. For chronic poor circulation it may be taken two or three times a day, for two to seven days, or until desired results are reached. For some, once or twice a week can be beneficial.

Contains: B complex, calcium, iron, manganese, and potassium.

CIRCULATION

*Blue Vervain

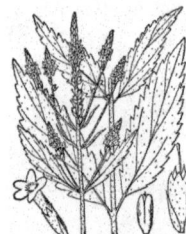

BLUE VERVAIN can be great for treating poor circulation. It is one of the best known herbs for treating poor circulation. Blue Vervain is a tonic that offers energy and fights fatigue. It gives a calming and tranquilizing effect to the system. **Large amounts of this herb taken at once may cause vomiting.** It may be taken in capsules. If it is taken as a tea, use ¼ teaspoon of Blue Vervain herb powder to one cup of boiling water. Blue Vervain may be taken as often as you feel the need. For chronic poor circulation it may be taken two or three times a day until desired results are reached. For some, once or twice a week will be beneficial.

Contains: vitamin C, calcium, manganese, and vitamin E.

Butcher's Broom

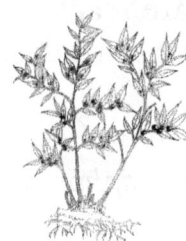

BUTCHER'S BROOM can be helpful for treating circulation; it offers circulation to the brain and veins. It prevents blood clots and leg cramps. It removes inflammation from the system. Butcher's Broom works great for people that must stand a lot. It may be taken in capsules. If it is taken as a tea, use ¼ teaspoon of Butcher's Broom herb powder to one cup of boiling water. Butcher's Broom may be taken as often as you feel the need. For poor circulation it may be taken two or three times a day for two to seven days, or until desired results are reached. For some, once or twice a week will be beneficial.

Contains: vitamins A, B1, B2, C, sodium, iron, potassium, calcium, niacin, selenium, and manganese.

CIRCULATION

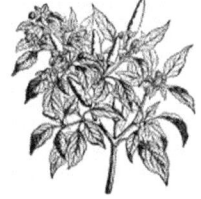

Capsium/Cayenne

CAPSICUM/CAYENNE affects the entire body for treating circulation; it is great for treating fatigue and excellent for treating varicose veins. It has a hot peppery taste and may be used with other herbs. It may be taken in capsules. If it is taken as a tea, use 1/8th teaspoon of capsicum/cayenne herb powder to one cup of boiling water. Capsicum/Cayenne may be taken as often as you feel the need. For chronic poor circulation it may be taken two or three times a day, for two to five days, or until desired results are reached. For some, once or twice a week will be beneficial.

Herbs for your blood type: Capsicum/Cayenne is highly beneficial for people with blood type O. It is neutral for people with blood B and AB. People with blood type A should avoid this herb."

Contains: vitamins A, C, magnesium, and sulphur, and it is very high in iron, potassium, and calcium.

Catnip

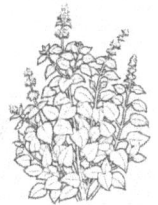

CATNIP will help to improve circulation; it reduces fatigue, it treats nausea and restlessness. It treats stress, hysteria, and helps to prevent miscarriage. It is a soothing herb and should be taken at bedtime. **Catnip may elevate blood pressure for some people when taken excessively.** Catnip may be taken in capsules. If it is taken as a tea, use ¼ teaspoon of Catnip herb powder to one cup of boiling water. Catnip may be taken as often as you feel the need. For poor circulation it may be taken two or three times a day, for two to seven days, or until desired results are reached. For some, once or twice a week will be beneficial.

Herbs for your blood type: Catnip is neutral for people with blood type O, B, and AB. People with blood type A should avoid this herb.

Contains: sodium, magnesium, iron, potassium, silicon, selenium, sulphur, and is rich in vitamins A, B complex, and C.

CIRCULATION

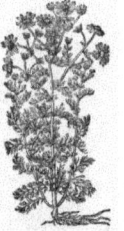

*Chamomile

CHAMOMILE can be great for treating poor circulation. It treats blood disorders, gangrene, and pain. Chamomile will relax an upset stomach and will increase the appetite. It may be taken in capsules. If it is taken as a tea, use ¼ teaspoon of Chamomile herb powder to one cup of boiling water. Chamomile may be taken as often as you feel the need. For chronic poor circulation it may be taken two or three times a day, for two to seven days, or until desired results are reached. For some, once or twice a week will be beneficial.

Herbs for your blood type: Chamomile is highly beneficial for people with blood type A and AB. It is neutral for people with blood type O, and B.

Contains: potassium, calcium, iron, manganese, vitamin A, and zinc.

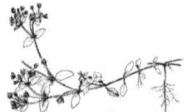

Chickweed

CHICKWEED will help with treating poor circulation. It removes plaque from the blood. It treats cancerous tumors, and cellulite. Chickweed will suppress the appetite. **Chickweed may elevate blood pressure for some people when taken excessively at once.** It may be taken in capsules. If it is taken as a tea, use ¼ teaspoon of Chickweed herb powder to one cup of boiling water. Chickweed may be taken as often as you feel the need. For poor circulation it may be taken once or twice a day, for two to five days, or until desired results are reached. For some, once or twice a week will be beneficial.

Herbs for your blood type: Chickweed is highly beneficial for people with blood type O. It is neutral for people with blood type A, B, and AB.

Contains sodium, zinc, and B complex, and is high in iron, vitamin C, minerals, calcium, and copper.

CIRCULATION

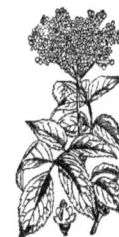

*Dong Quai

DONG QUAI is an excellent herb for treating poor circulation. It lubricates the intestines and purifies the blood. It treats chills, cancer, hot flashes, and a prolapsed uterus. Dong Quai may be taken in capsules. If it is taken as a tea, use ¼ teaspoon of Dong Quai herb powder to one cup of boiling water. Dong Quai may be taken as often as you feel the need. For chronic poor circulation it may be taken two or three times a day, for two to five days, or until desired results are reached. For some, once or twice a week will be beneficial.

Herbs for your blood type: Dong Quai is neutral for people with blood type O, A, B and AB.

Contains: vitamins A, B12 and E, and is very high in iron.

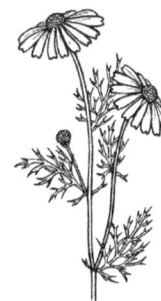

Feverfew

FEVERFEW will help to improve circulation. It treats rheumatoid arthritis and migraine headaches. It reduces inflammation and swelling. **Feverfew may elevate blood pressure for some people when taken excessively.** Feverfew may be taken in capsules. If it is taken as a tea, use ¼ teaspoon of Feverfew herb powder to one cup of boiling water. Feverfew may be taken as often as you feel the need. For poor circulation it may be taken two or three times a day for two to five days, or until desired results are reached. For some, once or twice a week will be beneficial for two to three weeks.

Contains: sodium, iron, niacin, potassium, selenium, zinc, and vitamins A and C.

CIRCULATION

*Garlic

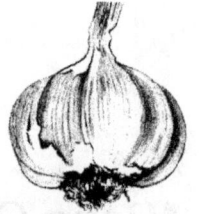

GARLIC can be great for improving circulation. It treats the lungs, asthma, and it improves arthritis. It is great for treating chronic bronchitis, and digestive disorders. **Garlic may elevate blood pressure for some people when taken excessively.** It may be taken in capsules. If it is taken as a tea, use ¼ teaspoon of Garlic herb powder to one cup of boiling water. Garlic may be taken as often as you feel the need. For chronic poor circulation it may be taken two or three times a day, for two to ten days, or until desired results are reached. For some, once or twice a week will be beneficial.

Herbs for your blood type: Garlic is highly beneficial for people with blood type A and AB. It is neutral for people with blood type O and B.

Contains: sodium, sulphur, calcium, copper, vitamin B1, iron, and is high in potassium, zinc, selenium, and vitamins A and C.

Gentian Root

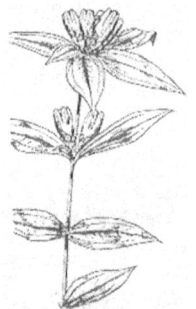

GENTIAN ROOT will assist with increasing circulation. It stimulates and strengthens the digestive system. It can be helpful with reducing fevers. It stimulates the pancreas and treats inflammation. Gentian will stimulate the appetite. It may be taken in capsules. If it is taken as a tea, use ¼ teaspoon of Gentian herb powder to one cup of boiling water. Gentian may be taken as often as you feel the need. For poor circulation it may be taken once or twice a day, for two to five days, or until desired results are reached. For some, once a week will be beneficial.

Contains: sulphur, tin, lead, manganese, zinc, niacin, and is high in iron.

CIRCULATION

*Ginger Root

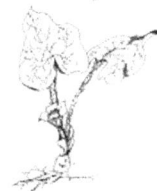

GINGER ROOT is great for stimulating circulation, especially for the feet and hands. It reduces fatigue, treats digestive disorders, and settles the stomach. It may be taken in capsules. If it is taken as a tea, use ¼ teaspoon of Ginger herb powder to one cup of boiling water. Ginger may be taken as often as you feel the need. For chronic poor circulation it may be taken two or three times a day until desired results are reached. For some, once or twice a week will be beneficial.

   Herbs for your blood type: Ginger is highly beneficial for people with blood type O, A, B and AB.

Contains: vitamins A, B complex, and C, calcium, iron, sodium, potassium, and magnesium.

*Ginkgo

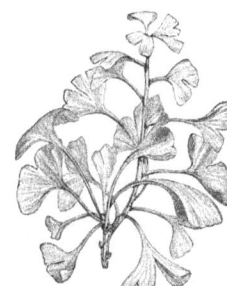

GINKGO is excellent for treating circulation. It treats circulatory disorders throughout the body, and helps to improve circulation in the auditory system. It improves mental clarity for Alzheimer's disease.. It improves oxygen flow to the brain, and will help with the prevention of strokes. It is an antioxidant, antiseptic stimulant. Ginkgo may be taken in capsules. If it is taken as a tea, use ¼ teaspoon of Ginkgo herb powder to one cup of boiling water. Ginkgo may be taken as often as you feel the need. For chronic poor circulation it may be taken two or three times a day, for two to seven days, or until desired results are reached. For some, once or twice a week will be beneficial.

Contains bioflavonoids

CIRCULATION

HERBS:

*Golden Seal

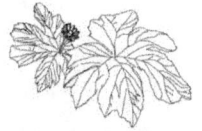

GOLDEN SEAL is among the best herbs for treating poor circulation. It treats infections, internal bleeding, and colds. Golden Seal will reduce sugar in the blood when it is used in combination with the Licorice herb. Use Myrrh with Golden Seal if there is a low blood sugar. **Do not take this herb if you are pregnant. Golden Seal may elevate blood pressure for some people.** Golden Seal may be taken in capsules. If it is taken as a tea, use ¼ teaspoon of Golden Seal herb powder to one cup of boiling water. Golden Seal may be taken as often as you feel the need. For chronic poor circulation it may be taken once or twice a day, for two to seven days, or until desired results are reached. For some, once or twice a week will be beneficial.

Herbs for your blood type: Golden Seal is neutral for people with blood type A, B and AB. People with blood type O should avoid this herb it will over stimulate the immune system and cause a blood thinning problem for blood type O.

Contains: sodium, calcium, potassium, iron, zinc, and vitamins A, C, B complex, and E.

Guggul

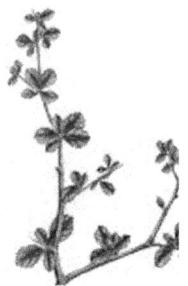

GUGGUL will help with circulation. It is best known for raising HDL cholesterol and lowering LDL cholesterol. It has a stimulating effect on the thyroid, and the heart. It may be taken in capsules. If it is taken as a tea, use ¼ teaspoon of Guggul herb powder to one cup of boiling water. Guggul may be taken as often as you feel the need. For poor circulation it may be taken once or twice a day, for two to five days, or until desired results are reached. For some, once or twice a week can be beneficial.

Content: vitamin information unknown.

CIRCULATION

HERBS:

*Horseradish

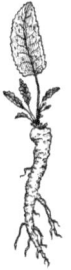

HORSERADISH can be highly beneficial for treating poor circulation; it treats rheumatism, digestive disorders, and asthma. Horseradish will stimulate the appetite. **Horseradish may elevate blood pressure for some people when taken excessively.** It may be taken in capsules. If it is taken as a tea, use ¼ teaspoon of Horseradish herb powder to one cup of boiling water. Horseradish may be taken as often as you feel the need. For chronic poor circulation it may be taken two or three times a day, for two to seven days, or until desired results are reached. For some, once or twice a week will be beneficial.

Contains: potassium, sulphur, sodium, iron, B complex, and it is high in vitamin C.

Licorice Root

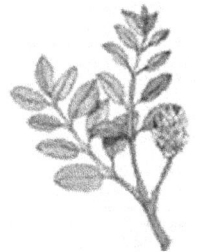

LICORICE ROOT is great for treating poor circulation. It strengthens the circulatory system, and reduces fatigue. It increases energy and it adds to longevity. Licorice will elevate blood sugar and cleanse the blood. **Licorice may elevate blood pressure for some people when taken excessively.** It is a bitter herb and it may be taken in capsules. If it is taken as a tea, use ¼ teaspoon Licorice herb powder to one cup of boiling water. Licorice may be taken as often as you feel the need. For chronic poor circulation it may be taken two or three times a day, for two to seven days, or until desired results are reached. For some, once or twice a week will be beneficial. .

Herbs for your blood type: Licorice is highly beneficial for people with blood type B and AB. It is neutral for people with blood type O and A.

Contains: niacin, lecithin, iodine, chromium, zinc, and vitamins E and B complex.

CIRCULATION

HERBS:

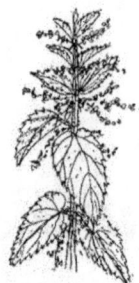

Nettles

NETTLES will help to increase poor circulation. It will assist with treating arthritis and gout. Nettles are an excellent source of minerals. It may be taken during pregnancy. It treats internal bleeding and urinary infections. Nettles will increase urine flow and act as a tonic for the hair. It may be taken in capsules. If it is taken as a tea, use ¼ teaspoon of Nettles herb powder to one cup of boiling water. Nettles may be taken as often as you feel the need. For poor circulation it may be taken once or twice a day, for two to five days, or until desired results are reached. For some, once or twice a week will be beneficial.

Contains: calcium, chlorophyll, chromium, copper, iron, manganese, potassium, protein, silicon, sodium, sulphur, and vitamins A, C, D, E, F, and P, and zinc.

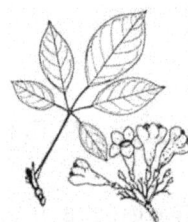

Pau D' Arco

PAU D'ARCO helps to eliminate poor circulation. It removes age spots from the body. It will boost immune system and help to relieve pain caused by cancer. It is very high in iron. Pau D'Arco may be taken in capsules. If this herb is taken as a tea, use ¼ teaspoon of Pau D'Arco herb powder to one cup of boiling water. Pau D'Arco may be taken as often as you feel the need. For poor circulation it may be taken once or twice a day, for two to five days, or until desired results are reached. For some, once or twice a week will be beneficial.

Contains: potassium, sodium, magnesium, manganese, selenium, zinc, and vitamins A, B complex, and C, and is very high in iron.

CIRCULATION

*Pine Tree Bark

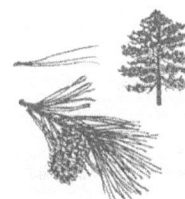

PINE TREE BARK is an excellent choice for treating poor circulation. It treats varicose veins, phlebitis, heart disease and arthritis. It may be taken in capsules. If it is taken as a tea, use ¼ teaspoon of Pine Tree Bark herb powder to one cup of boiling water. Pine Tree Bark may be taken as often as you feel the need. For chronic poor circulation it may be taken once or twice a day, for two to five days, or until desired results are reached. For some, once or twice a week will be beneficial.

Contains: bioflavonoids and vitamin C.

*Prickly Ash

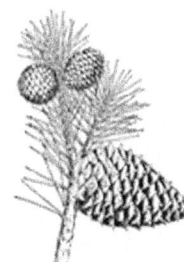

PRICKLY ASH is great for treating circulation; it works throughout the vascular system. It helps with treating problems in the joints. It treats varicose veins and increases the flow of saliva in the mouth. It treats a wide variety of conditions. It warms cold hands, cold feet, and cold legs. It may cause some people to become more sensitive to sunlight and burn more easily. It helps to treat yeast growth and gonorrhea. It may be taken in capsules. If it is taken as a tea, use ¼ teaspoon of Prickly Ash herb powder to one cup of boiling water. Prickly Ash may be taken as often as you feel the need. For chronic poor circulation it may be taken once or twice a day, for two to ten days, or until desired results are reached. For some, once or twice a week will be beneficial.

Contains tannins.

CIRCULATION

Rosemary

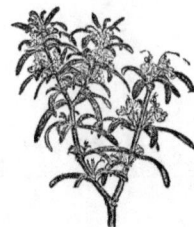

ROSEMARY can be very effective for treating poor circulation. It treats stress, tension, and depression. When Rosemary is used with Myrrh it will stop bleeding gums. It may be taken in capsules. If it is taken as a tea, use ¼ teaspoon of Rosemary herb powder to one cup of boiling water. Rosemary may be taken as often as you feel the need. For poor circulation it may be taken two or three times a day for two to five days, or until desired results are reached. For some, once or twice a week will be beneficial.

Contains: iron, sodium, potassium, zinc, phosphorus, magnesium, vitamins A and C, and is high in calcium.

Sage

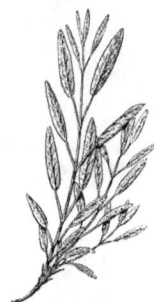

SAGE can be helpful for treating poor circulation. It improves the memory, and is a hair tonic that treats baldness. It treats nausea and nervous conditions. Sage will dry up saliva, perspiration, and mother's milk after birth. Sage may be used in the kitchen as a spice. Sage may be taken in capsules. When it is taken as a tea use ¼ teaspoon of Sage herb powder to one cup of boiling water. Sage may be taken as often as you feel the need. For poor circulation it may be taken two or three times a day for two to seven days, or until desired results are reached. For some, once or twice a week will be beneficial.

Herbs for your blood type: Sage is highly beneficial for people with blood type B. It is neutral for people with blood type O, A, and AB.

Contains: sodium, sulphur, vitamins A, B complex, and C.

CIRCULATION

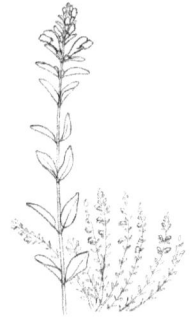

Skullcap

SKULLCAP will help to treat poor circulation. It soothes the nerves and detoxifies severe withdrawals of alcohol addiction and tremors. Skullcap may elevate blood pressure for some people when taken excessively. Skullcap may be taken in capsules. If it is taken as a tea, use ¼ teaspoon of Skullcap herb powder to one cup of boiling water. Skullcap may be taken as often as you feel the need. For poor circulation it may be taken two or three times a day for two to seven days, or until desired results are reached. For some, once or twice a week will be beneficial.

Herbs for your blood type: Skullcap is neutral for people with blood type O and A. People with blood type B and AB should avoid this herb.

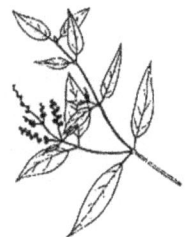

*Suma

SUMA is excellent for treating chronic circulation; it strengthens the immune system. It treats cancer, cholesterol, and it offers vitality to the body. Suma may be taken in capsules. If it is taken as a tea, use ¼ teaspoon of Suma herb powder to one cup of boiling water. Suma may be taken as often as you feel the need. For chronic poor circulation it may be taken two or three times a day, for two to five days, or until desired results are reached. For some, once or twice a week will be beneficial.

Contains: iron, magnesium, vitamin B complex, minerals, and amino acids.

COLON

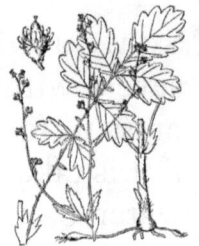

Agrimony

AGRIMONY offers nutrients that will treat the colon; it treats, stomach cancer, colitis, kidney stones, and liver disorders. It treats bladder problems and uterine bleeding. It is excellent for treating jaundice and skin diseases. Agrimony is a tonic and it maybe taken in capsules. If it is taken as a tea, use ¼ teaspoon of Agrimony herb powder to one cup of boiling water. Agrimony may be taken as often as you feel the need. For treating the colon it may be taken once or twice a day, for five to seven days, or until the desired results are reached. For some, once or twice a week can be beneficial.

Contains: iron, niacin, vitamin K, and B3.

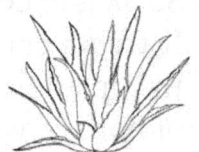

Aloe

ALOE can offer assistance for treating the colon. It treats colitis problems, it will sooth the stomach, and treat allergy problems. Aloe has also been known to act as a buffer against proliferation of the HIV virus. Aloe may be taken in capsules. When it is taken as a tea use ¼ teaspoon of Aloe herb powder to one cup of boiling water. Aloe may be taken as often as you feel the need. For treating the colon it may be taken once or twice a day, for three to five days, or until the desired results are reached. For some, once or twice a week can be beneficial.

COLON

Herbs for your blood type: Aloe is highly beneficial for people with blood type A. People with blood type O, B and AB should avoid using this herb. as much as possible internally.

Contains: potassium, sodium, manganese, iron, and zinc.

Basil

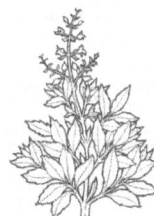

BASIL will help to treat the colon; it treats stomach cramps and spasms. It can be effective for promoting and stimulating energy. Some herbalists recommend it for lowering cholesterol and triglyceride levels. Basil may be taken in capsules. If it is taken as a tea, use ¼ teaspoon of Basil herb powder to one cup of boiling water. Basil may be taken as often as you feel the need. For treating the colon it may be taken once or twice a day, for three to five days, or until desired results are reached. For some, once or twice a week can be beneficial.

Herbs for your blood type: Basil is neutral for people with blood type O, A, B, and AB.

Contains: iron, calcium, magnesium, phosphorus, and vitamins A, D, and B2.

Bayberry

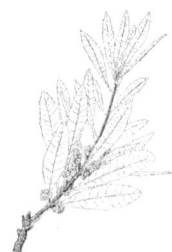

BAYBERRY can be a good remedy for treating the colon; it treats the stomach, diarrhea and excessive menstrual bleeding. It offers vitality to the body. Bayberry is a tonic. It may be taken in capsules. If it is taken as a tea, use ¼ teaspoon of Bayberry herb powder to one cup of boiling water. Bayberry may be taken as often as you feel the need. For colon problems it may be taken once or twice a day, for two to five days, or until desired results are reached. For some, once or twice a week can be beneficial.

Contains: calcium, sodium, magnesium, manganese, niacin, potassium, silicon, phosphorus, zinc, vitamins B1, B2, and C.

COLON

HERBS:

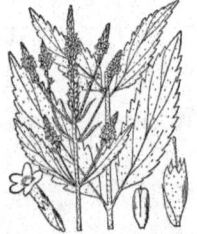

*Blue Vervain

BLUE VERVAIN will truly settle the stomach and quiet the colon; it gives a calm and tranquilizing effect on the system. It treats poor circulation, insomnia, toxic liver problems and nervous disorders. **Large amounts of Blue Vervain taken at once may cause vomiting.** It is a pleasant tasting herb and it may be taken in capsules. If it is taken as a tea, use ¼ teaspoon of Blue Vervain herb powder to one cup of boiling water. Blue Vervain may be taken as often as you feel the need. For severe colon problems it may be taken once or twice a day, for two to seven days, or until desired results are reached. For some, once or twice a week can be beneficial.

Contains: vitamin C, calcium, manganese, and vitamin E.

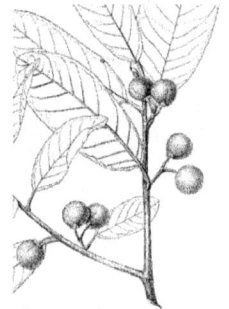

Cascara Sagrada

CASCARA SAGRADA will clean and restore order to the colon. It treats chronic problems such as colitis, constipation, and stomach disorders. Cascara Sagrada is a bitter herb and it may be taken in capsules. If it is taken as a tea, use ¼ teaspoon of Cascara Sagrada herb powder to one cup of boiling water. Cascara Sagrada may be taken as often as you feel the need. For colon problems it may be taken once or twice a day, for three to seven days, or until desired results are reached. For some, once or twice a week can be beneficial.

Contains: calcium, potassium, B complex, manganese, lead, aluminum, and tin.

COLON

Chamomile

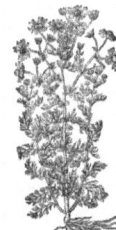

CHAMOMILE will help to settle the colon. It will quiet the stomach when you suffer cramps. Chamomile treats colitis, colic, and nervous disorders. It will also increase the appetite. It may be taken in capsules, if it is taken as a tea, use ¼ teaspoon of Chamomile herb powder to one cup of boiling water. Chamomile may be taken as often as you feel the need. For treating the colon it may be taken once or twice a day, for two to seven days, or until the desired results are reached. For some, once or twice a week can be beneficial.

Herbs for your blood type: Chamomile is highly beneficial for people with blood type A and AB. It is neutral for people with blood type O, and B.

Contains: potassium, calcium, iron, manganese, vitamins A, and zinc.

Chaparral

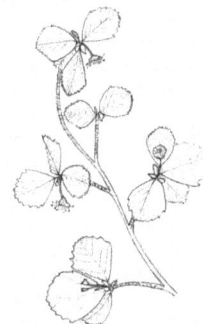

CHAPARRAL is a good remedy for the colon; it treats stomach disorders and cramps. It will help to prevent these problems when taken periodically. It may be taken in capsules. If it is taken as a tea, use ¼ teaspoon of Chaparral herb powder to one cup of boiling water. Chaparral may be taken as often as you feel the need. For treating the colon it may be taken once or twice a day, for five to seven days, or until the desired results are reached. For some, once or twice a week can be beneficial for two to three weeks.

Contains: sodium, potassium, aluminum, barium, chlorine, protein, silicon, and sulphur.

COLON

HERBS:

Chickweed

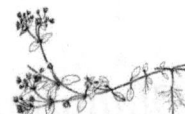

CHICKWEED can be included for treating the colon; it treats colitis, and restores tissue lining to the stomach. Chickweed will suppress the appetite. **Chickweed may elevate blood pressure for some people when taken excessively.** It may be taken in capsules. If it is taken as a tea, use ¼ teaspoon of Chickweed herb powder to one cup of boiling water. Chickweed may be taken as often as you feel the need. For treating the colon it may be taken once or twice a day for five to seven days, or until desired results are reached. For some, once or twice a week can be beneficial.

Herbs for your blood type: Chickweed is highly beneficial for people with blood type O. It is neutral for people with blood type A, B, and AB.

Contains: sodium, zinc, and B complex, and is high in iron, vitamin C, minerals, calcium, and copper.

Cloves

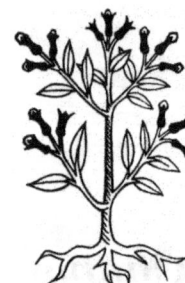

CLOVES can be a good choice for treating the colon; it treats colitis, treats bad breath, and increases circulation of the blood. It helps to relieve nausea when taken as a tea. It may be taken in capsules. If Cloves is taken as a tea, use ¼ teaspoon of Cloves herb powder to one cup of boiling water. Cloves may be taken as often as you feel the need. For colon problems it may be taken once or twice a day, for five to seven days, or until desired results are reached. For some, once or twice a week can be beneficial.

Contains: sodium, potassium, calcium, magnesium, phosphorus, vitamins A, B complex, and C.

COLON

Comfrey

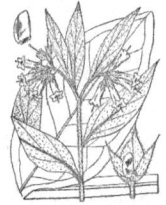

COMFREY treats inflammation of the colon; it treats colitis, cancer, stomach disorder, and the entire pancreas. Comfrey may be taken in capsules, if it is taken as a tea use ¼ teaspoon of Comfrey herb powder to one cup of boiling water. Comfrey may be taken as often as you feel the need. For colon problems it may be taken once or twice a day, for five to seven days, or until desired results are reached. For some, once or twice a week can be beneficial.

Contains: vitamins A, C, iron, sulphur, copper, zinc, and magnesium. Comfrey is very high in calcium, potassium, and protein.

Dandelion

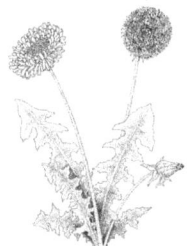

DANDELION will assist with treating the colon; it treats the stomach, cramps, and pancreas problems. **Dandelion may elevate blood pressure for some people when taken excessively.** Dandelion may be taken in capsules. If it is taken as a tea, use ¼ teaspoon of Dandelion herb powder to one cup of boiling water. Dandelion may be taken as often as you feel the need. For colon problems it may be taken once or twice a day, for three to four days, or until desired results are reached. For some, once or twice a week can be beneficial.

Herbs for your blood type: Dandelion is highly beneficial for people with blood type O. It is Neutral for people with blood type A, B, and AB.

Contains: calcium, vitamin A, B, C, and E, sodium, potassium, iron, nickel, tin, copper, magnesium, manganese, sulphur, and zinc.

COLON

Fennel

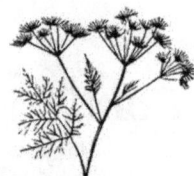

FENNEL can be helpful with treating the colon, it treats acid in the stomach, and most intestinal problems. It will lower cholesterol. **Fennel may elevate blood pressure for some people when taken excessively.** Fennel may be kept in the kitchen and used a spice. Fennel may be taken in capsules. If it is taken as a tea, use ¼ teaspoon of Fennel herb powder to one cup of boiling water. Fennel may be taken as often as you feel the need. For treating the colon it may be taken once or twice a day, for three to five days, or until desired results are reached. For some, once or twice a week can be beneficial.

Contains: sodium, potassium and sulphur and is high in vitamin A.

*Garlic

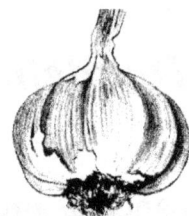

GARLIC is very effective for treating the colon. It treats colitis when used as an enema or colonic. It will rid the colon of parasites. It treats fungus and poor circulation. **Garlic may elevate blood pressure for some people when taken excessively.** It may be taken in capsules. If it is taken as a tea, use ¼ teaspoon of Garlic herb powder to one cup of boiling water. Garlic may be taken as often as you feel the need. For severe colon problems it may be taken once or twice a day for three to five days or until desired results are reached. For some, one or twice a week can be beneficial.

Herbs for your blood type: Garlic is highly beneficial for people with blood type A and AB. It is neutral for people with blood type O and B.

Contains: sodium, sulphur, calcium, copper vitamin B1, and iron, and is high in potassium, zinc, selenium, and vitamins A and C.

COLON

HERBS:

*Ginger

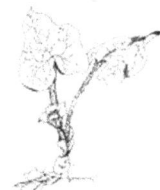

GINGER is great for treating inflammation of the colon; it treats colon spasms, and cramps. Do not take aspirins while using Ginger; it will inhibit the performance of the herb. It may be taken in capsules. If it is taken as a tea, use ¼ teaspoon of Ginger herb powder to one cup of boiling water. Ginger may be taken as often as you feel the need. For severe colon problems it may be taken once or twice a day, for three to seven days, or until desired results are reached. For some, one or twice a week can be beneficial.

Herbs for your blood type: Ginger is highly beneficial for people with blood type O, A, B and AB.

Contains: vitamins A, B complex, C, calcium, iron, sodium, potassium, and magnesium.

*Golden Seal

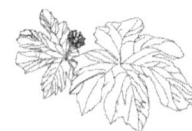

GOLDEN SEAL can be very effective for treating the colon; it treats inflammation of the colon and chronic stomach problems. Golden Seal will reduce sugar in the blood when it is used with the licorice herb. Use Myrrh with Golden Seal if you suffer low blood sugar. **Do not take this herb if you are pregnant. Golden Seal may elevate blood pressure for some people when taken excessively.** It may be taken in capsules. If it is taken as a tea, use ¼ teaspoon of Golden Seal herb powder to one cup of boiling water. Golden Seal may be taken as often as you feel the need. For severe colon problems it may be taken once or twice a day, for five to seven days, or until desired results are reached. For some, once or twice a week can be beneficial.

Herbs for your blood type: Golden Seal is neutral for people with blood type A, B and AB. People with blood type O should avoid this herb it will over stimulate the immune system and cause a blood thinning problem for blood type O.

Contains: sodium, calcium, potassium, iron, zinc, and vitamins A, C, B complex, and E.

COLON
---

*Kelp

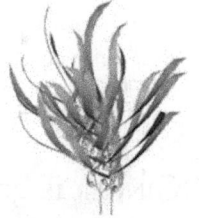

KELP can be an excellent choice for treating the colon. It treats colitis and it removes lead from the body. Kelp affects the thyroid by balancing an overactive, or under active thyroid gland. Kelp will promote healthy hair growth. It may be taken in capsules. If it is taken as a tea, use ¼ teaspoon of Kelp herb powder to one cup of boiling water. Kelp may be taken as often as you feel the need. For severe colon problems it may be taken once or twice a day, for two to five days, or until the desired results are reached. For some, once or twice a week can be beneficial.

Contains: calcium, chlorine sulphur, silicon, zinc, manganese, aluminum, potassium, copper, nickel, iron, silver, phosphorus, vanadium, B complex, vitamins A, C, E, and K, has is very high content of iodine, and minerals.

Myrrh

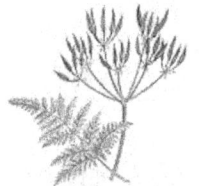

MYRRH will help to cleanse the colon, it treat colitis. It is a stimulant that brings order to the entire system. Myrrh will stimulate and promote menstruation. Myrrh has antiseptic properties and it may be used in place of Golden Seal. Myrrh may be taken in capsules. When it is taken as a tea use ¼ teaspoon of Myrrh herb powder to one cup of boiling water. Myrrh may be taken as often as you feel the need. For the colon it may be taken once or twice a day, for two to seven days, or until the desired results are reached. For some, once or twice a week can be beneficial.

Contains: potassium, sodium, chlorine, silicon, and zinc.

COLON

Pau D'Arco

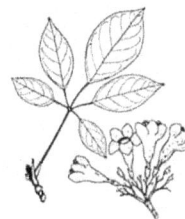

PAU D'ARCO helps to clean the colon; it will assist with treating colitis problems. Pau D'Arco will increase red corpuscles. It has many virus killing powers. It may be taken in capsules. If it is taken as a tea, use ¼ teaspoon of Pau D'Arco herb powder to one cup of boiling water. Pau D'Arco may be taken as often as you feel the need. For colon problems it may be taken once or twice a day, for two to five days, or until the desired results are reached. For some, once or twice a week can be beneficial.

Contains: potassium, sodium, magnesium, manganese, selenium, and zinc. Vitamins A, B complex and C and is very high in iron.

*Peppermint

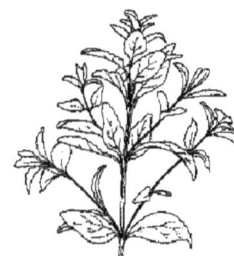

PEPPERMINT is an excellent herb to use for the colon. It treats colitis and offers relief for stomach spasms and nausea. It may be taken in capsules. If it is taken as a tea, use ¼ teaspoon of Peppermint herb powder to one cup of boiling water. Peppermint may be taken as often as you feel the need. For colon problems it may be taken once or twice a day, for two to seven days, or until the desired results are reached. For some, once or twice a week can be beneficial.

Herbs for your blood type: Peppermint is highly beneficial for people with blood type O and B. It is neutral for people with blood type A and AB.

Contains: iron, niacin, iodine, magnesium, sulphur, potassium, and vitamins A and C.

COLON

Plantain

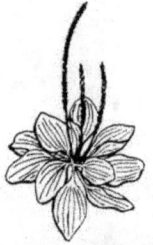

PLANTAIN will help to treat the colon. It treats colitis, neutralizes stomach acid, and will help with mild stomach ulcers. It helps to remove toxins from the bowels. It acts as a mild laxative and will ease the pain. Plantain will suppress the appetite and it lowers cholesterol. Plantain is not the same as the Plantain fruit fount in the produce section of the market. Plantain may be taken in capsules, if it is taken as a tea, use ¼ teaspoon of Plantain herb powder to one cup of boiling water. Plantain may be taken as often as you feel the need. For colon problems it may be taken once or twice a day for two to seven days, or until the desired results are reached. For some, once or twice a week can be beneficial.

Contains: a high amount of vitamins C and K, calcium, sulphur, potassium, and minerals.

*Psyllium

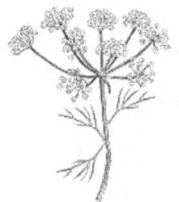

PSYLLIUM is excellent for cleaning the colon; it treats colitis, constipation and irritable bowel syndrome. It is excellent for treating diverticulitis. It may be taken in capsules. If it is taken as a tea, use ¼ teaspoon of Psyllium herb powder to one cup of boiling water. Psyllium may be taken as often as you feel the need. For cleaning the colon it may be taken once or twice a day, for three to five days, or until desired results are reached. For some, once or twice a week can be beneficial.

Content: vitamin information unknown.

COLON

HERBS:

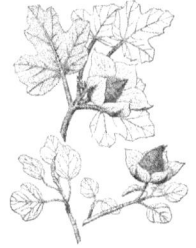

Slippery Elm

SLIPPERY ELM is an excellent choice for cleaning the colon; it treats colitis, gastrointestinal problems, stomach problems and ulcers. Slippery Elm should be taken in capsules because it will not dissolve in liquid. Slippery Elm may be taken as often as you feel the need. For colon problems it may be taken once or twice a day until the desired results are reached. For some, once or twice a week can be beneficial.

Herbs for your blood type: Slippery Elm is highly beneficial for people with blood type O, and A. It is neutral for people with blood type B and AB.

Contains: iron, sodium, iodine, zinc, copper, potassium, and vitamins K and E.

DIABETES

*Alfalfa

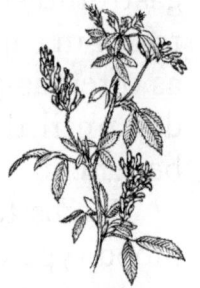

ALFALFA can be great for treating diabetes. It treats urinary problems, contaminated kidneys, acidity, nosebleeds, and nausea. Alfalfa may be taken in capsules. If it is taken as a tea use ¼ teaspoon of Alfalfa herb powder to one cup of boiling water, Alfalfa may be taken as often as you feel the need. For diabetes it may be taken once or twice a day, for two to seven days, or until desired results are reached. For some once or twice a week for three to four weeks can be beneficial.

Herbs for your blood type: Alfalfa is highly beneficial for people with blood type A. It is neutral for people with blood type B and AB. People with blood type O should avoid this herb it will cause excessive blood thinning for them.

Contains: vitamins A, B complex, D, E, and K, iron, potassium, magnesium, protein, sodium, sulfur, and phosphorus, and is very high in calcium, chlorophyll, and vitamin B12.

DIABETES

Astragalus

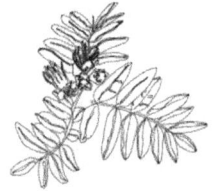

ASTRAGALUS can be helpful with treating diabetes. It strengthens the digestion system, improves circulation, lowers blood pressure, and strengthens T-cells. Urination will increase while using this herb. Astragalus may be taken in capsules. If it is taken as a tea, use ¼ teaspoons of Astragalus herb powder to one cup of boiling water. Astragalus may be taken as often as you feel the need. For diabetes it may be taken once or twice a day, for two to seven days, or until desired results are reached. For some, once or twice a week for three to four weeks can be helpful.

Contains: choline, betaine, and gluconic acid.

Barley Juice Powder

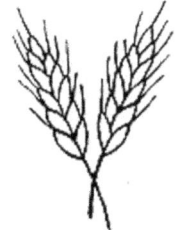

BARLEY JUICE POWDER can be helpful for treating diabetes; it treats kidney problems, cancer, high blood pressure, and it will reduce fever. It may be taken in capsules. If it is taken as a tea, use ¼ teaspoon of Barley Juice Powder to one cup of boiling water. Barley Juice Powder may be taken as often as you feel the need. For diabetes it may be taken once or twice a day, for two to seven days, or until desired results are reached. For some, once or twice a week can be helpful.

Contains: vitamins B1, B12, and C, potassium, and iron, and is high in calcium.

DIABETES

HERBS:

*Bilberry

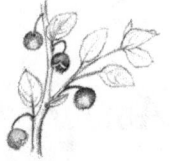

BILBERRY can be very effective for treating diabetes. It treats urinary problems, as well as bladder and kidney infections. Bilberry will increase night vision. It can be helpful during pregnancy to strengthen the veins. Bilberry may be taken in capsules. If it is taken as a tea, use 1/8th teaspoon of Bilberry herb powder to one cup of boiling water. Bilberry may be taken as often as you feel the need. For diabetes, it may be once or twice a day, for two to seven days, or until desired results are reached. For some, two or three times a week for two or three weeks can be helpful.

Contains: manganese, iron, zinc, potassium, calcium, sodium, and selenium.

*Blue Cohosh

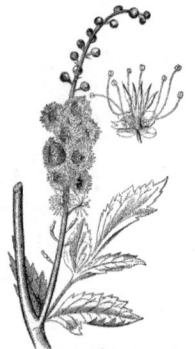

BLUE COHOSH can be excellent for treating diabetes. It's great for treating urinary infections and inflammation. Blue Cohosh will induce labor and should not be used by pregnant women until the ninth month. It helps with treating toxemia. Blue Cohosh is a diuretic. It may be taken in capsules. If it is taken as a tea, use 1/8th teaspoon of Blue Cohosh to one cup of boiling water. Blue Cohosh may be taken as often as you feel the need. For diabetes it may be taken once or twice a day, for five to seven days, or until desired results are reached. For some two or three times a week for three or four weeks can be beneficial.

Contains: vitamin E, calcium, B complex, potassium, phosphorus, and magnesium.

DIABETES

Buchu

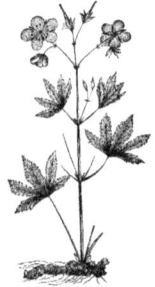

BUCHU can be helpful to use for early stages of diabetes; it treats inflammation of the kidneys and urinary problems. Urination will increase while using Buchu. It will reduce irritation in the bladder. It may be taken in capsules. If it is taken as a tea, use ¼ teaspoon of Buchu herb powder to one cup of boiling water. Buchu may be taken as often as you feel the need. For diabetes it may be taken two or three times a week for two or three weeks for desired results.

Contains bioflavonoids.

Bugleweed

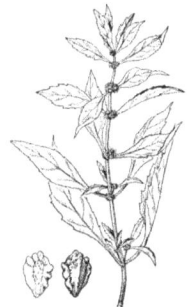

BUGLEWEED will be helpful with treating diabetes. It treats urinary problems, overactive thyroid problems, calms the heart, and eases pain. Bugleweed will lower the pulse rate and stabilize irregular heartbeats. It treats palpitations and a weak heart due to edema. It may be taken in capsules. If it is taken as a tea, use ¼ teaspoon of Bugleweed herb powder to one cup of boiling water. Bugleweed may be taken as often as you feel the need. For diabetes it may be taken once or twice a day, for three to seven days, or until desired results are reached, for some, two or three times a week can be helpful.

Content: vitamin information unknown.

DIABETES

HERBS:

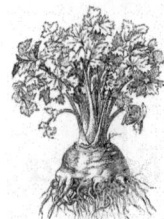

Celery

CELERY can helpful for treating diabetes. It will increase urine flow. Celery will remove arthritis and gout from the system. It produces a calming effect on the system. It may be taken in capsules. If it is taken as a tea, use ¼ teaspoon of Celery herb powder, to one cup of boiling water. Celery herb powder may be taken as often as you feel the need. For diabetes it may be taken once or twice a day, for three to seven days, or until desired results are reached. For some, two or three times a week can be helpful.

Contains: potassium, calcium, iron, magnesium, sulfur, vitamins A, B, and C, organic sodium, and is high in iron.

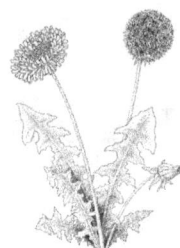

Dandelion

DANDELION will assist with treating diabetes; it offers relief for urinary and kidney problems. It detoxifies poisons from the liver, treats gout, and water retention. Dandelion may elevate blood pressure for some people when taken excessively. Dandelion may be taken in capsules. If it is taken as a tea, use ¼ teaspoon of Dandelion herb powder to one cup of boiling water. Dandelion may be taken as often as you feel the need. For diabetes it may be taken once or twice a day, for three to seven days, or until desired results are reached. For some, two or three times a week will be helpful for desired relief.

Herbs for your blood type: Dandelion is highly beneficial for people with blood type O. It is neutral for people with blood type A, B, and AB.

Contains: calcium, vitamin A, B, C, E, sodium, potassium, iron, nickel, tin, copper, magnesium, manganese, sulphur, and zinc.

DIABETES

*Devil's Claw

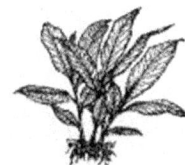

DEVIL'S CLAW is a great herb for treating diabetes. It strengthens chronic bladder and kidney problems, treats hardening of the arteries, gout, and pain inthe joints. Devil's Claw may be taken in capsules. If it is taken as a tea, use ¼ teaspoon of Devil's Claw herb powder to one cup of boiling water. Devil's Claw may be taken as often as you feel the need. For diabetes it may be taken once or twice a week for desired results.

Contains: sodium, potassium, calcium, protein, iron, silicon, selenium, phosphorus, zinc, and vitamins A and C.

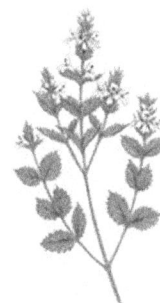

*Eyebright

EYEBRIGHT will treat chronic diabetes. It helps to clean the blood, and it is stimulating to the liver. It is great for improving eye problems. It has strong antiseptic properties and will treat an earache like no other herb can. Eyebright may be taken in capsules. If it is taken as a tea, use ¼ teaspoon of Eyebright herb powder to one cup of boiling water. Eyebright may be taken as often as you feel the need. For diabetes it may be taken two or three times a week until desired results are reached.

Contains: vitamins D, E, B complex, iron, iodine, copper, and zinc.

DIABETES

HERBS:

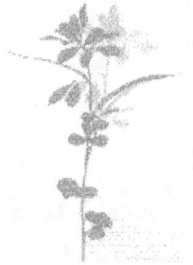

*Fenugreek

FENUGREEK can be extremely helpful for treating diabetes. It helps to treat kidney problems, and will help to reduce urinary glucose levels. It helps to clean the lymphatic system, and it treats water retention. Fenugreek should not be used by women who wish to get pregnant, it will impede the progress. It may be taken in capsules. If it is taken as a tea, use ¼ teaspoon of Fenugreek herb powder to one cup of boiling water. Fenugreek may be taken as often as you feel the need. For diabetes it may be taken two or three times a week until desired results are reached.

Herbs for your blood type: Fenugreek is highly beneficial for people with blood type O, and A. People with blood type B, or AB should avoid this herb.

Contains: vitamins B1, B2, iron, and choline, and is very rich in vitamins A and D.

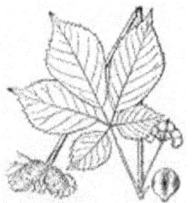

*Gingseng/Panax

GINSENG/PANAX is a terrific herb to use for treating diabetes; it stimulates the appetite and provides energy to the body. Long-term use is not recommended for women, it will produce testosterone, which will increase hormones. Two weeks on and four weeks off will do fine for women. Ginseng/Panax herb will benefit men on long term just great! This herb is better prepared in glass cookware, as metal pots will reduce the strength. It may be taken in capsules, if it is taken as a tea, use ¼ teaspoon Ginseng/Panax herb powder to one cup of boiling water. Ginseng/Panax may be taken as often as you feel the need. For diabetes it may be taken two or three times a week until desired results are reached.

Herbs for your blood type: Ginseng is highly beneficial for Blood types O, A, B, and AB.

DIABETES

Contains: vitamins A, B12, and E, iron, calcium, magnesium, sodium, sulphur, niacin, potassium, silicon, manganese, and phosphorus.

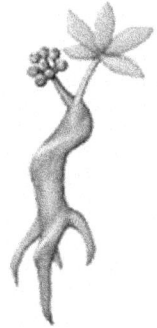

Ginseng/Siberian

GINSENG/SIBERIAN will help with treating diabetes. It offers endurance, longevity and helps with memory problems. It treats chronic anxiety and promotes speedy recover after surgery. It may be taken in capsules. If it is taken as a tea, use ¼ teaspoon of Ginseng/Siberian herb powder to one cup of boiling water. Ginseng/Siberian may be taken as often as you feel the need. For diabetes it may be taken two or three times a week until desired results are reached.

Contains: B12, sulphur, calcium, iron, sodium, and potassium.

*Horsetail

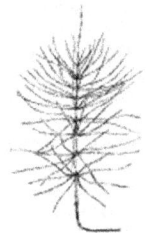

HORSETAIL can be an excellent treatment for diabetes. It clears up urinary problems just great! Horsetail stimulates hair growth and it stimulates circulation. It kills parasites, and keeps calcium in the body. It will increase urination. **Horsetail may elevate blood pressure for some people when a large amount is taken at once.** Horsetail may be taken in capsules. If it is taken as a tea, use ¼ teaspoon of Horsetail herb powder to one cup of boiling water. Horsetail may be taken as often as you feel the need. For diabetes it may be taken two or three times a week until desired results are reached.

Contains: sodium, iron, iodine, copper, vitamin E, and a high content of silicon and selenium.

DIABETES

HERBS:

*Juniper

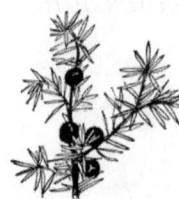

JUNIPER is a great herb to use for treating diabetes. It treats kidney and bladder infections. This herb produces natural insulin to the body. Juniper is not recommended for pregnant women. It may be taken in capsules. If it is taken as a tea, use ¼ teaspoon of Juniper herb powder to one cup of boiling water. Juniper may be taken as often as you feel the need. For diabetes it may be taken two or three times a week until desired results are reached.

Contains: sulphur, copper, and a small amount of aluminum, and a high amount of vitamin C.

Kelp

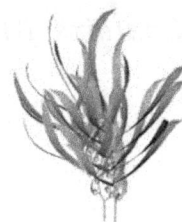

KELP will assist with the treatment of diabetes. It helps to regulate the kidneys, and it removes lead from the body. It will help with treating the bladder, prostate, and uterine difficulties. Kelp will affect the thyroid by balancing an overactive or under active thyroid gland. Kelp stimulates healthy hair growth. It may be taken in capsules. If it is taken as a tea, use ¼ teaspoon of Kelp herb powder to one cup of boiling water. Kelp may be taken as often as you feel the need. For diabetes it may be taken once a day for two to seven days, or until desires results are reached. For some, once or twice a week can be helpful.

Contains: iodine, calcium, chlorine sulphur, silicon, zinc, manganese, aluminum, potassium, copper, nickel, iron, silver, phosphorus, vanadium, B complex, vitamins A, C, E, and K, and a very high content of iodine and minerals.

HERBS:

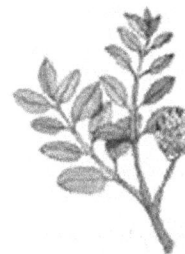

*Licorice

LICORICE can be very beneficial for treating diabetes. It raises blood sugar levels to normal levels. It treats Addison's disease, increases energy, treats weight loss, and gastrointestinal problems. Use potassium with this herb. Licorice will elevate high blood pressure when used in large amounts. It may be taken in capsules. If it is taken as a tea, use ¼ teaspoon of Licorice herb powder to one cup of boiling water. Licorice may be taken as often as you feel the need. For diabetes it may be taken once or twice a week until desired results are reached.

Herbs for your blood type: Licorice is highly beneficial for people with blood type B and AB. It is neutral for people with blood type O and A.

Contains: niacin, lecithin, iodine, chromium, zinc, and vitamins E and B complex.

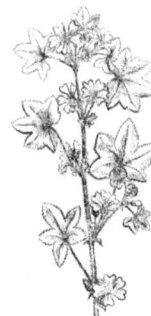

Marshmallow

MARSHMALLOW helps with treating diabetes. It offers a soothing effect on the system and the urinary problems that accompany diabetes. **Marshmallow may elevate blood pressure for some people when taken excessively at once.** Marshmallow may be taken in capsules. If it is taken as a tea, use ½ teaspoon of Marshmallow herb powder to one cup of boiling water. Marshmallow may be taken as often as you feel the need. For diabetes it may be taken once or twice a day, for two to seven days, or until desired results are reached. For some, once or twice a week can be helpful.

Do not confuse Marshmallow with the candy like marshmallow found in the food section of the market.

Contains: sodium, iodine, B complex, pantothenic acid, and is high in calcium, zinc, and iron.

DIABETES

HERBS:

Oregon Grape

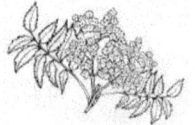

Oregon Grape can be useful for treating diabetes. It stimulates the liver and cleans the blood. It has been known to have a stimulating effect on the thyroid. It stimulates the appetite and purifies the blood. This is a great herb to take in place of Golden Seal. It cleans the liver organs, and will increase the strength of the immune system and helps to relieve constipation. It may be taken in capsules. If it is taken as a tea use ¼ teaspoon of Oregon Grape herb powder to one cup of boiling water. Oregon Grape may be taken as often as you feel the need. For treating diabetes it may be taken once a day for two to seven days or until desired results are reached. For some once or twice a week can be helpful.

Contains: sodium, zinc, manganese, copper, and silicon.

*Pau D'Arco

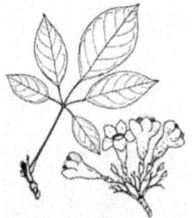

Pau D'Arco can be very beneficial for treating diabetes. It has been known to lower dependence on insulin injections. It purifies the blood, assists with the treatment of AIDS, herpes, and other venereal diseases. It relieves prostate problems. Pau D'Arco may elevate blood pressure for some people when a large amount is taken at once. Pau D'Arco is a bitter herb and it may be taken in capsules. If it is taken as a tea, use ¼ teaspoon of Pau D'Arco herb powder to one cup of boiling water. Pau D'Arco may be taken as often as you feel the need. For diabetes it may be taken once a day until desired results are reached. For some, once or twice a week can be beneficial.

Contains: potassium, sodium, magnesium, manganese, selenium, zinc vitamins A, B complex, and C, and is very high in iron.

DIABETES

HERBS:

Periwinkle

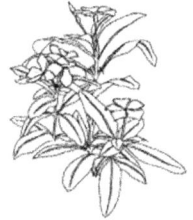

PERIWINKLE benefits the entire system while treating diabetes; it helps to improve the kidneys, liver, and lungs. It treats cancer, Hodgkin's disease, and strengthens the lymphatic system. Periwinkle calms the nervous system and lowers blood pressure. Periwinkle is a sedative. Periwinkle will protect brain cells and increase oxygen flow to the brain. It helps to reduce brain injury after strokes. It may be taken in capsules. If it is taken as a tea, use ½ teaspoon of Periwinkle herb powder to one cup of boiling water. Periwinkle may be taken as often as you feel the need. For diabetes it may be taken once a day for two to five days, or until desired results are reached. For some, once a week can be beneficial.

Do not over use.

Content: vitamin information unknown.

*Pine Tree Bark

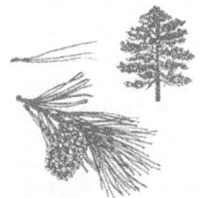

PINE TREE BARK can be very beneficial for treating diabetes. It helps to improve the vascular system, the retina, blindness, and it helps to improve night vision. It treats cancer, phlebitis, and stress. Pine Tree Bark may be taken in capsules. If it is taken as a tea, use ¼ teaspoon of Pine Tree Bark herb powder to one cup of boiling water. Pine Tree Bark may be taken as often as you feel the need. For diabetes it may be taken once or twice a day until desired results are reached. For some, two or three times a week can be beneficial.

Contains vitamin C.

DIABETES

HERBS:

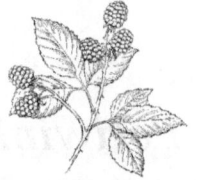

Red Raspberry

RED RASPBERRY will assist with the treatment of diabetes. It cleans and purifies the blood. Red Raspberry helps to relieve painful childbirth; it strengthens the uterus, and stops morning sickness. Red Raspberry treats AIDS and the prostate gland. It may be taken in capsules. If it is taken as a tea, use ¼ teaspoon of Red Raspberry herb powder to one cup of boiling water. Red Raspberry may be taken as often as you feel the need. For diabetes it may be taken once or twice a day until desired results are reached. For some, two or three times a week can be beneficial.

Contains: calcium, manganese, vitamins A, B, C, D, and E. Red Raspberry is very high in iron.

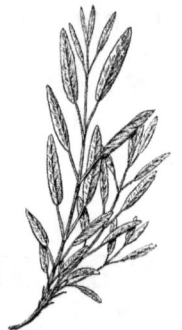

*Sage

SAGE can be excellent for treating diabetes; it treats poor circulation, and bleeding problems. Sage will help to prevent baldness, it stops coughs, lowers fevers, and improves memory loss. It stops nausea and eliminates night sweats. Sage may elevate blood pressure in some people when taken excessively. Sage may be taken in capsules. If it is taken as a tea, use ½ teaspoon of Sage herb powder to one cup of boiling water. Sage may be taken as often as you feel the need. For diabetes it may be taken once or twice a day until desired results are reached. For some, two or three times a week can be beneficial.

Herbs for your blood type: Sage is highly beneficial for people with blood type B. It is neutral for people with blood type O, A, and AB.

Contains: sodium, sulphur, vitamins A, B complex, and C.

DIABETES

HERBS:

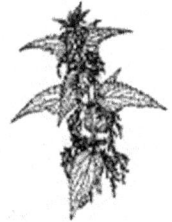

Saw Palmetto

SAW PALMETTO will help to treat diabetes. It will correct urinary problems and treat bladder diseases. It reduces an enlarged prostate, and eliminates impotency. Saw Palmetto is a sexual stimulant. It may be taken in capsules. If it is taken as a tea use ½ teaspoon of Saw Palmetto herb powder to one cup of boiling water. Saw Palmetto may be taken as often as you feel the need. For diabetes it may be taken once or twice a day until desired results are reached. For some, two or three times a week can be beneficial.

Contains vitamin A.

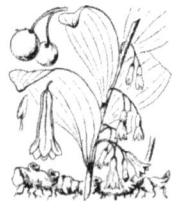

*Schizandra

SCHIZANDRA can be great for treating diabetes. Schizandra will increase urination; it increases energy, gives mental alertness and eliminates impotency. Schizandra may elevate blood pressure for some people when used excessively. It may be taken in capsules. If it is taken as a tea, use ½ teaspoon of Schizandra herb powder to one cup of boiling water. Schizandra may be taken as often as you feel the need. For diabetes it may be taken once or twice a day until desired results are reached. For some, two or three times a week can be beneficial.

Contains: magnesium, calcium, iron, vitamin C, potassium, and sodium.

DIABETES

HERBS:

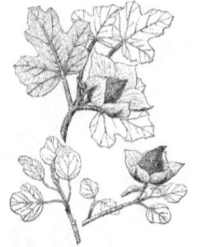

Slippery Elm

SLIPPERY ELM will help to treat diabetes. It treats bladder and urinary infections. It treats asthma, bronchitis and lung problems. Slippery Elm should be taken in capsules because it will not dissolve in liquid. Slippery Elm may be taken as often as you feel the need. For diabetes it may be taken once or twice a day until desired results are reached. For some, two or three times a week can be beneficial.

Herbs for your blood type: Slippery Elm is highly beneficial for people with blood type O, and A. It is neutral for people with blood type B and AB.

Contains: iron, sodium, iodine, zinc, copper, potassium, and vitamins K and E.

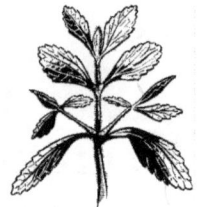

*Stevia

STEVIA can be a friend to diabetics. It is a sugar substitute that can be used as a sweetener: a very small amount goes a long way. It stops tobacco cravings and suppresses the appetite. For diabetics, it is said to be safe. Stevia herb powder may be taken in capsules. When it is taken as a tea, use 1/8th or less of Stevia herb powder to one cup of water. Stevia may be taken as often as you feel the need. For diabetes it may be taken once or twice a day until desired results are reached. For some, two or three times a week can be beneficial.

Herbs for your blood type: Stevia is neutral for people with blood types O, A, B and AB.

Contains: vitamins A, iron, potassium, selenium, silicon, sodium, niacin, and zinc.

DIABETES

*Uva Ursi

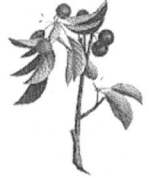

UVA URSI is an excellent for treating diabetes. Uva Ursi clears up urinary problems, eliminates kidney infections, treats venereal diseases and it strengthens heart muscles. **Do not use this herb during pregnancy it will cause damage to the fetus. Uva Ursi increases the flow of urine and acts as a disinfectant.** Uva Ursi will turn the urine a dark green do not panic, it is normal. Uva Ursi may be taken in capsules. If it is taken as a tea, use ¼ teaspoon of Uva Ursi to one cup of boiling water. Uva Ursi may be taken as often as you feel the need. For diabetes it may be taken once or twice a day, for two to ten days, or until desired results are reached. For some, two or three times a week can be beneficial.

Contains: iron, manganese, trace minerals, and vitamin A.

DIGESTIVE DISORDERS

HERBS:

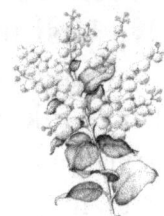

Acacia

ACACIA will soothe an irritated digestive tract. It treats inflammation in the system and the mucous membranes. It helps to soothe the stomach, bowels, uterus, and vaginal area. It is helpful with treating sore throats and diarrhea. Acacia may be taken in capsules. If it is taken as a tea, use ¼ teaspoon of Acacia herb powder to one cup of boiling water. Acacia may be taken as often as you feel the need. For digestive disorders it may be taken once or twice a day, for three to seven days, or until desired results are reached. For some, once or twice a week can offer desired results.

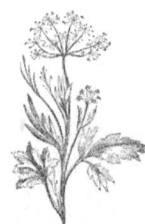

*Anise

ANISE is a great herb for treating digestive disorders. It treats indigestion, prevents fermentation in the system, and it treats gas. It stimulates the appetite, and can be stimulating to vital organs such as the heart, liver, lungs and brain. It has high estrogen levels and Anise may be used as a spice in the kitchen. Anise may be taken in capsules. If it is taken as tea, use ½ teaspoon of Anise herb powder to one cup of boiling water. Anise may be taken as often as you feel the need. For treating chronic digestive disorders it may be taken once or twice a day, for three to seven days, or until desired results are reached. For some, once or twice a week can be beneficial.

Contains: iron, calcium, potassium, magnesium, and B vitamins.

DIGESTIVE DISORDERS

HERBS:

*Barberry

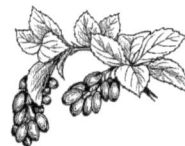

BARBERRY is excellent for treating digestive disorders. It treats chronic indigestion and stimulates the appetite. Barberry treats liver problems, mouth ulcers, and syphilis. It dilates blood vessels, which assists with lowering blood pressure. **Do not take Barberry excessively it may cause depression.** It may be taken in capsules, if it is taken as a tea, use ¼ teaspoon of Barberry herb powder to one cup of boiling water. Barberry may be taken as often as you feel the need. For chronic digestive disorders it may be taken once or twice a day for three to seven days, or until desired results are reached. For some once or twice a week can offer results.

Contains: iron, manganese, phosphorus, and vitamin C .

*Bayberry

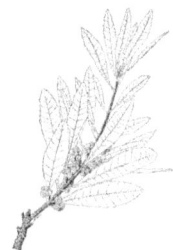

BAYBERRY can be very effective for treating digestive disorders. It offers relief from indigestion, and is a tonic that offers vitality to the body. It may be taken in capsules. If it is taken as a tea, use ½ teaspoon of Bayberry herb powder to one cup of boiling water. Bayberry may be taken as often as you feel the need. For chronic digestive disorders it may be taken once or twice a day, for two to five days, or until desired results are reached. For some, once or twice a week can be effective.

Contains: calcium, sodium, magnesium, manganese, niacin, potassium, silicon, phosphorus, zinc, vitamins B1, B2, and C.

DIGESTIVE DISORDERS

Bee Pollen

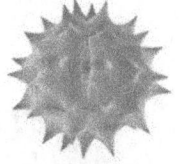

BEE POLLEN will assist with treating digestive disorders. It treats indigestion and will stimulate the appetite. It treats exhaustion, restores energy, offers longevity, and treats early stages of multiple sclerosis. It is best to begin taking small amounts of this herb in the beginning and increase it as your system adjusts to it. It rejuvenates the whole body as it builds the blood. It may be taken in capsules. If it is taken as a tea, use ½ teaspoon of Bee Pollen herb powder to one cup of boiling water. Bee Pollen may be taken as often as you feel the need. For digestive disorders and indigestion it may be taken once or twice a day, for two to five days, or until desired results are reached. For some, once or twice a week can be helpful for prevention.

Contains: vitamin C, B complex, enzymes, iron, magnesium, manganese, potassium, sodium, and amino acids.

Bee's Royal Jelly

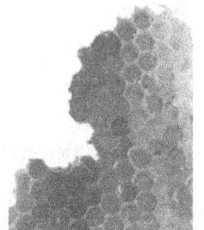

BEE'S ROYAL JELLY can be helpful for treating digestive disorders. It increases energy, boosts the immune system, and it treats prostate problems. It may be taken in capsules. If it is taken as a tea, use ¼ teaspoon of Bee's Royal Jelly herb powder to one cup of boiling water. Bee's Royal Jelly may be taken as often as you feel the need. For digestive disorders it may be taken once or twice a day, for three to seven days, or until desired results are reached. For some, once or twice a week can be helpful for desired results.

Bee's Royal Jelly is high in all of the B vitamins, and in minerals.

DIGESTIVE DISORDERS

HERBS:

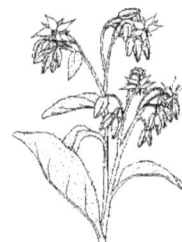

Borage

BORAGE can be a good choice for treating the digestive system. It strengthens the heart and acts as a tonic for the entire body. It treats bronchitis, and is excellent for treating eye inflammation. Borage is a bitter herb and it may be taken in capsules. If it is taken as a tea, use ¼ teaspoon of Borage herb powder to one cup of boiling water. Borage may be taken as often as you feel the need. For digestive disorders it may be taken once or twice a day, for three to seven days, or until desired results are reached. For some, once or twice a week can be helpful for desired results.

Contains: calcium and potassium.

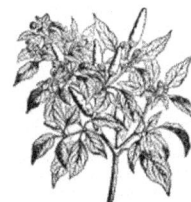

*Capiscum/Cayenne

CAPSICUM/CAYENNE will treat digestion disorders; it treats indigestion, inflammation, and jaundice. It is great for treating infections and shock. It is a hot and spicy herb and may be used in combination with other herbs. It may be taken in capsules. When it is taken as a tea, use 1/8th teaspoon or less of Capsicum/Cayenne herb powder to one cup of boiling water. Capsicum/Cayenne may be taken as often as you feel the need. For digestive disorders it may be taken once or twice a day, for three to seven days, or until desired results are reached. For some, once or twice a week can offer desired results

Herbs for your blood type: Capsicum/Cayenne is highly beneficial for people with blood type O. It is neutral for people with blood type B and AB. People with blood type A should avoid this herb.

Contains: vitamins A, C, magnesium, and sulphur. Capsicum/Cayenne is very high in iron, potassium, and calcium.

DIGESTIVE DISORDERS

HERBS:

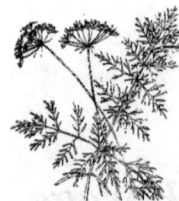

*Caraway

CARAWAY can be excellent for treating digestive disorders. It settles the stomach, relieves spasms, acid, and treats menstrual cramps. Caraway will stimulate the appetite. It may be taken in capsules, if it is taken as a tea, use 1/8th teaspoon of Caraway herb powder to one cup of boiling water. Caraway may be taken as often as you feel the need. For chronic digestive disorders it may be taken once or twice a day, for three to seven days, or until desired results are reached. For some, once or twice a week can give results.

Contains: calcium, potassium, copper, iodine, iron, lead, magnesium, silicon, cobalt, zinc, and vitamin B complex

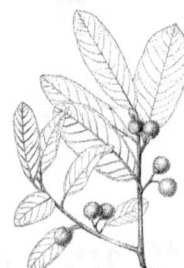

Cascara Sagrada

CASCARA SAGRADA can be effective for treating digestive disorders. It treats indigestion, cleans toxic bowel matter from the system, and cleans the colon. It helps to lower blood pressure. Cascara Sagrada may be taken in capsules. If it is taken as a tea, use ½ teaspoon of Cascara Sagrada herb powder to one cup of boiling water. **Cascara Sagrada should be taken with a pinch of Kelp or burdock added.** It may be taken as often as you feel the need. For digestive disorders it may be taken once a day for two to five days, or until desired results are reached. For some, once or twice a week can be beneficial.

Contains: calcium, potassium, vitamin B complex, manganese, lead, aluminum, and tin.

DIGESTIVE DISORDERS

HERBS:

Catnip

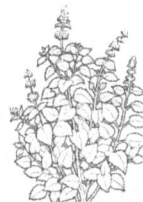

CATNIP will assist with treating digestive disorders. It treats indigestion, convulsions, hysteria, insanity, **and** spasms. It will improve circulation. Catnip may be taken in capsules. If it is taken as a tea, use ¼ teaspoon of Catnip herb powder to one cup of boiling water. Catnip may be taken as often as you feel the need. For digestive disorders it may be taken once or twice a day, for two to five days, or until desired results are reached. For some, once or twice a week can offer desired results.

Herbs for your blood type: Catnip is neutral for people with blood type O, B, and AB. People with blood type A should avoid this herb.

Contains: magnesium, sodium, iron, potassium, silicon, selenium, sulphur, and is high in vitamins A, B complex, and C.

*Centaury

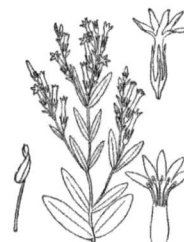

CENTAURY is an ancient herb that strengthens the digestive system. It stimulates the appetite and purifies the blood. **Pregnant women should not use Centaury; it will not be safe for a developing baby.** This herb may be taken in capsules. If it is taken as a tea, use ¼ teaspoon of Centaury herb powder to one cup of boiling water. Centaury may be taken as often as you feel the need. For chronic digestive problems it may be taken once or twice day for three to five days, or until desired results are reached. For some, once or twice a week can be beneficial.

DIGESTIVE DISORDERS

HERBS:

*Chicory

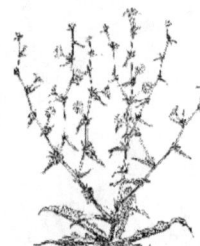

CHICORY is excellent for treating chronic digestion disorders; It's great for treating stiff joints, and it helps to remove calcium deposits from the system. It purifies the blood. It may be taken in capsules. If it is taken as a tea, use ¼ teaspoon of Chicory herb powder to one cup of boiling water. Chicory may be taken as often as you feel the need. For chronic digestive disorders it may be taken once or twice day for two to five days, or until desired results are reached. For some, once or twice a week offers benefit.

Contains: a high amount of vitamins A, B, C, K and P.

*Cinnamon

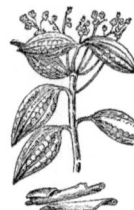

CINNAMON can be excellent for treating digestive disorders. It treats gas, nausea, cancer, rheumatism, vomiting, chest discomfort, and indigestion. Cinnamon may cause excessive menstrual flow. **Pregnant women should avoid Cinnamon during pregnancy. Men with prostate problems should avoid Cinnamon. Diabetics should consult a health care provider before taking Cinnamon: some herbalists say it will increase insulin activity.** Cinnamon may be used as a spice in the kitchen. It may be taken in capsules. If it is taken as a tea, use ¼ teaspoon of cinnamon herb powder to one cup of boiling water. Cinnamon may be taken as often as you feel the need. For chronic digestive disorders it may be taken once or twice a day for three to seven days, or until desired results are reached. For some, once or twice a week can be beneficial.

Herbs for your blood type: Cinnamon is neutral for people with blood type A and blood type AB. People with blood type O and blood type B should avoid this herb.

Contains: calcium, chromium, copper, iodine, manganese, potassium, zinc, tannin, B-vitamins, vitamins A and C.

DIGESTIVE DISORDERS

Comfrey

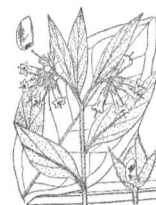

COMFREY can be useful for treating the digestive system. It is soothing and repairs the respiratory system. Comfrey stimulates new cell growth; provides healing, and promotes healthy skin. It may be taken in capsules. If it is taken as a tea, use ¼ teaspoon of Comfrey herb powder to one cup of boiling water. Comfrey may be taken as often as you feel the need. For chronic digestive disorders it may be taken once or twice day for two to five days, or until desired results are reached. For some, once or twice a week can be beneficial.

Contains: vitamins A, C, iron, sulphur, copper, zinc and magnesium. Comfrey is very high in calcium, potassium, and protein.

Dandelion

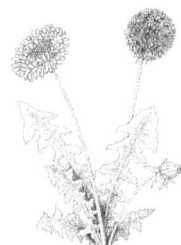

DANDELION will help with treating digestive disorders. It also lowers cholesterol, and helps to remove stiffness in the joints. It increases urine flow. **Dandelion may elevate blood pressure for some people when taken excessively.** Dandelion may be taken in capsules. If it is taken as a tea, use ¼ teaspoon of Dandelion herb powder to one cup of boiling water. Dandelion may be taken as often as you feel the need. For digestive disorders it may be taken once or twice a day, for two to five days, or until desired results are reached. For some, once or twice a week will give desired relief.

Herbs for your blood type: Dandelion is highly beneficial for people with blood type O. It is neutral for people with blood type A, B, and AB.

Contains: calcium, vitamin A, B, C, E, sodium, potassium, iron, nickel, tin copper magnesium, manganese, sulphur, and zinc, and is high in nutrients.

DIGESTIVE DISORDERS

HERBS:

Elder Flower

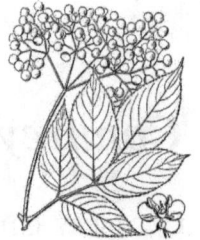

ELDER FLOWER will assist with treating digestive disorders. It is an anti- inflammatory agent and is very useful for treating bronchitis and circulation of the blood. Elder Flower will promote sweating. It's good for treating the lungs and asthma. It may be taken in capsules. If it is taken as a tea, use ¼ teaspoon of Elder Flower herb powder to one cup of boiling water. Elder Flower may be taken as often as you feel the need. For digestive disorders it may be taken once or twice a day, for three to seven days, or until desired results are reached. For some, once or twice a week can be helpful.

Contains: vitamins A and C.

Elecampane

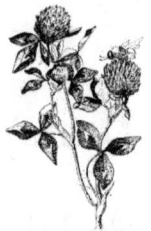

ELECAMPANE will assist with treating digestive disorders. It will increase the appetite and lower blood sugar levels. It will reduce water retention. Elecampane may be used in combination with other herbs. It may be taken in capsules. If it is taken as a tea, use ¼ teaspoon of Elecampane herb powder to one cup of boiling water. Elecampane may be taken as often as you feel the need. For digestive disorders it may be taken once or twice a day for two to five days, or until desired results are reached. For some, once or twice a week can be beneficial for prevention.

Contains: sodium, calcium, and potassium.

DIGESTIVE DISORDERS

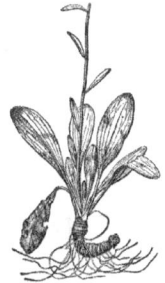

*False Unicorn

FALSE UNICORN is an excellent choice to use for digestive disorders. It will strengthen the reproductive organs and it increases urine flow. It is best known for its treatment of the prostate and prolapsed uterus problems. It may be taken in capsules. If it is taken as a tea, use ¼ teaspoon of False Unicorn herb powder to one cup of boiling water. False Unicorn may be taken as often as you feel the need. For chronic digestive disorders it may be taken once or twice a day until desired results are reached. For some, once or twice a week can be beneficial.

Contains: vitamin C, sulphur, copper, cobalt, cadmium, and zinc.

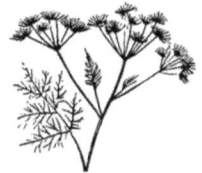

*Fennel

FENNEL will improve sluggish digestion disorders. It is excellent for treating indigestion problems. It expels gas, and reduces acid in the stomach. It works well with other herbs and will curb the appetite. It treats intestinal problems and it works great for treating morning sickness. It will lower cholesterol. Fennel may elevate blood pressure for some people when used excessively. Fennel can be used as a spice. Fennel may be taken in capsules. If it is taken as a tea, use ½ teaspoon of Fennel herb powder to one cup of boiling water. Fennel may be taken as often as you feel the need. For chronic digestive disorders it may be taken once or twice a day, for two to seven days, or until desired results are reached. For some, once or twice a week will be beneficial.

Contains: sodium, potassium, and sulphur, and is high in vitamin A.

DIGESTIVE DISORDERS

HERBS:

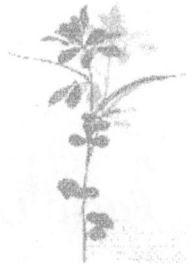

*Fenugreek

FENUGREEK is great for treating digestive disorders. It treats stomach irritations and inflamed intestines. For treating allergies it is a must-have. Fenugreek should not be used by women who wish to get pregnant, it will impede the progress. Fenugreek may be taken in capsules. If it is taken as a tea, use ¼ teaspoon of Fenugreek herb powder to one cup of boiling water. Fenugreek may be taken as often as you feel the need. For chronic digestive disorder it may be taken once or twice a day, for two to five days, or until desired results are reached. For some, once or twice a week, can offer relief for prevention.

Herbs for your blood type: Fenugreek is highly beneficial for people with blood type O, and A. People with blood type B, or AB should avoid this herb.

Contains: B1, B2, iron, and choline, and is very rich in vitamins A and D.

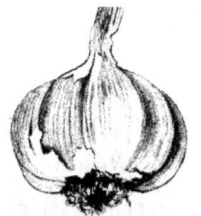

*Garlic

GARLIC can be great for treating digestive disorders. It will stimulate circulation, treat chronic bronchitis, and purify the blood. **Garlic may elevate blood pressure for some people when taken excessively.** Garlic may be taken in capsules. If it is taken as a tea, use ¼ teaspoon of Garlic herb powder to one cup of boiling water. Garlic may be taken as often as you feel the need. For chronic digestive disorder it may be taken once or twice day for two to seven days, or until desired results are reached. For some, once or twice a week can be beneficial.

Herbs for your blood type: Garlic is highly beneficial for people with blood type A and AB. It is neutral for people with blood type O and B.

Contains: sodium, sulphur, calcium, copper vitamin B1, and iron, and is high in potassium, zinc, selenium, and vitamins A and C.

DIGESTIVE DISORDERS

HERBS:

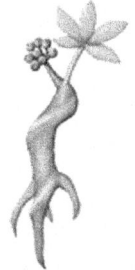

Ginseng/Siberian

GINSENG/SIBERIAN will help to treat digestive disorders. It treats poor circulation, protects from radiation, and increases mental alertness. **Ginseng/Siberian may elevate blood pressure for some people when taken excessively.** If it must be taken, it should be used in combination with other herbs, and used not more than once a week: use only a small pinch of the Ginseng/Siberian. It may be taken in capsules. If it is taken as a tea, use ¼ teaspoon of Ginseng Siberian herb powder to one cup of boiling water. Ginseng/Siberian may be taken as often as you feel the need. For digestive disorders it may be taken once or twice a day, for two to five days, or until desired results are reached. For some, once or twice a week can be helpful.

Contains: B12, sulphur, calcium, iron, sodium, and potassium.

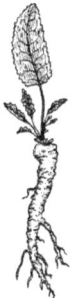

*Horsedish

HORSERADISH will stimulate the digestive system. It stimulates the appetite, expels worms from the body, and increases circulation. **Horseradish may elevate blood pressure for some people when taken excessively.** If it must be taken, it should be used in combination with other herbs and use only a small pinch of the Horseradish. Horseradish may be taken in capsules. If it is taken as a tea, add ¼ teaspoon of Horseradish herb powder to one cup of boiling water. Horseradish may be taken as often as you feel the need. For chronic digestive problems it may be taken once or twice a day, for two to five days, or until desired results are reached. For some, once or twice a week can be beneficial until desired results are reached.

Contains: potassium, sulphur, sodium, iron, B complex, and is high in vitamin C.

DIGESTIVE DISORDERS

HERBS:

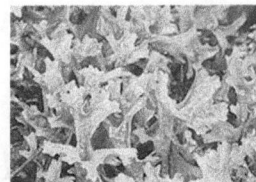

*Iceland Moss

ICELAND MOSS is excellent for treating digestive disorders. It treats the entire upper respiratory system including tuberculosis. Iceland Moss may be taken in capsules. If it is taken as a tea, use ¼ teaspoon of Iceland Moss herb powder to one cup of boiling water. Iceland Moss may be taken as often as you feel the need. For chronic digestive disorders it may be taken once or twice a day, for two to five days, or until desired results are reached. For some, once or twice a week for two to three weeks can be beneficial for prevention.

Contains: calcium, potassium, and iodine.

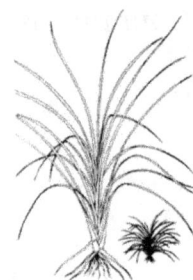

Lemon Grass

LEMON GRASS can be effective for treating digestive disorders. It will reduce mucus from the respiratory system, it treat asthma, indigestion, vomiting, colds, coughs, and flu. It will increase urination and help to treat internal parasites. Lemon Grass may be taken in capsules. If it is taken as a tea, use ¼ teaspoon of Lemon Grass herb powder to one cup of boiling water. Lemon Grass may be taken as often as you feel the need. For digestive disorders it may be taken once or twice a day, for two to five days, or until desired results are reached. For some, once or twice a week can be effective.

Contains: calcium, iron, magnesium, manganese, phosphorus, potassium, selenium, and zinc, and is high in vitamins A and C.

DIGESTIVE DISORDERS

HERBS:

Lobelia

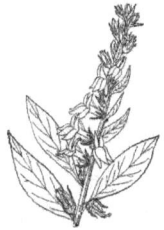

LOBELIA will help with treating digestive disorders. It will relax and sooth the entire respiratory system and it can be very effective in treating acute asthma and coughs. Lobelia will increases urine flow. It may be taken in capsules. If it is taken as a tea, use ¼ teaspoon of Lobelia herb powder to one cup of boiling water. Lobelia may be taken as often as you feel the need. For digestive disorders it may be taken once or twice a day, for two to five days, or until desired results are reached. For some, once or twice a week can be helpful for desired results.

Contains: iron, copper, sodium, sulphur, cobalt, lead, and selenium.

LOTS OF WATER SHOULD BE TAKEN WITH LOBELIA.

*Oregon Grape

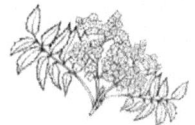

OREGON GRAPE is excellent for treating digestive disorders. It is an excellent herb for people that are unable to take Golden Seal. This herb will stimulate the thyroid functions. It cleans the liver organs, and increases the immune system. **Oregon Grape may elevate blood pressure for some people when taken excessively.** If it must be taken, it should be used it in combination with other herbs and use only a small pinch of the Oregon Grape. Oregon Grape may be taken in capsules. If it is taken as a tea, use ¼ teaspoon of Oregon Grape herb powder to one cup of boiling water. Oregon Grape may be taken as often as you feel the need. For digestive disorders it may be taken once or twice a day, for two or three days, or until desired results are reached. For some, once or twice a week can be useful.

Contains: sodium, zinc, manganese, copper, and silicon.

HERBS TO HELP YOU HEAL

| **DIGESTIVE DISORDERS** |

HERBS:

Parsley

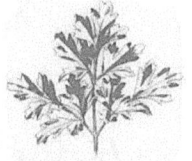

PARSLEY will help to relieve digestive disorders. It is excellent for cancer prevention when it is used in large amounts over a long period. It will sweeten the breath. **Use Parsley in moderation during pregnancy: it will induce labor pains.** However, after birth it will dry up mother's milk during the weaning period. It may be taken in capsules. If it is taken as a tea, use ¼ teaspoons of Parsley herb powder to one cup of boiling water. Parsley may be taken as often as you feel the need. For digestive disorders it may be taken two or three times a day for two to seven days, or until desired results are reached. For some, once or twice a week can be helpful.

Herbs for your blood type: Parsley is highly beneficial for people with blood type O and B. It is neutral for people with blood type A and AB.

Contains: vitamins A, B, and C, chlorophyll, iron, potassium, calcium, cobalt, copper, riboflavin, silicon, sodium, sulphur, and thiamine.

*Peppermint

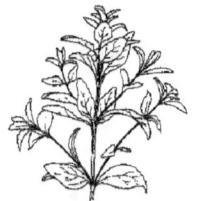

PEPPERMINT is highly recommended for treating digestive disorders. It treats heartburn, gas, and nausea. Peppermint may be taken in capsules. If this herb is taken as a tea, use ¼ teaspoon of Peppermint herb powder to one cup of boiling water. Peppermint may be taken as often as you feel the need. For digestive problems it may be taken once or twice a day, for two to seven days, or until desired results are reached. For some, once or twice a week can be excellent for results.

Herbs for your blood type: Peppermint is highly beneficial for people with blood type O and B. It is neutral for people with blood type A and AB.

Contains: iron, niacin, iodine, magnesium, sulphur, potassium, and vitamins A and C.

DIGESTIVE DISORDERS

Prickly Ash

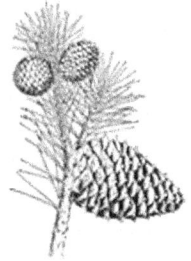

PRICKLY ASH treats a wide variety of conditions, including a weak digestive system. It will strengthen the digestive system and increase poor circulation. Prickly Ash will increase the flow of saliva in the mouth. It warms cold hands, cold feet, and cold legs. It may cause some people to become more sensitive to sunlight and burn more easily. It helps to treat yeast growth and gonorrhea. Prickly Ash can be taken in capsules. If it is taken as a tea, use ¼ teaspoon of prickly ash herb powder to one cup of boiling water. Prickly Ash may be taken as often as you feel the need. For digestive disorders it may be taken once or twice a day, for two to five days, or until desired results are reached. For some, once or twice a week can be beneficial.

Contains tannins.

*Red Raspberry

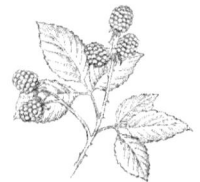

RED RASPBERRY is great for treating digestive disorders. Red Raspberry works best for mother during pregnancy and after childbirth. It enhances the production of milk in the breasts. Children may also use this herb for treating colds. It may be taken in capsules. If it is taken as a tea, use ½ teaspoon of Red Raspberry herb powder to one cup of boiling water. Red Raspberry may be taken as often as you feel the need. For chronic digestive disorders it can be taken once or twice a day, for two to five days, or until desired results are reached. For some, once or twice a week can be beneficial.

Contains: calcium, manganese, vitamins A, B, C, D, and E. Red Raspberry is very high in iron.

DIGESTIVE DISORDERS

HERBS:

*Safflower

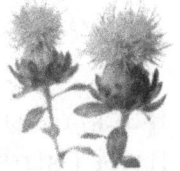

SAFFLOWER is excellent for treating digestive disorders; it is at the top for treatment and relief. It treats heartburn and stomach acid. It increases perspiration, and increases the flow of urine. Safflower stimulates the pancreas, clears phlegm from the lungs, and will produce temporary insulin. It may be taken in capsules. If it is taken as a tea, use ¼ teaspoon of Safflower herb powder to one cup of boiling water. Safflower may be taken as often as you feel the need. For chronic digestive disorders it can be taken once or twice a day, for two to five days, or until desired results are reached. For some, once or twice a week can be beneficial.

Contains vitamin K.

*Saffron

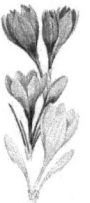

SAFFRON can be excellent treatment for digestive disorders. It improves circulation and offers energy to the system. It treats cancer, headaches, liver problems, and urinary problems. Saffron may be kept in the kitchen as used as a spice. It may be taken in capsules. If it is taken as a tea, use ¼ teaspoon of Saffron herb powder to one cup of boiling water. Saffron may be taken as often as you feel the need. For chronic digestive disorders it may be taken once or twice a day, for two to five days, or until desired results are reached. For some, once or twice a week can be beneficial. **Saffron may elevate blood pressure for some people when taken excessively.** If it must be taken, it should be used in combination with other herbs and use only a small pinch of the saffron.

Contains: sodium, calcium, potassium, and vitamins A and B 12.

DIGESTIVE DISORDERS

*Sage

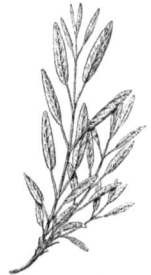

SAGE gives excellent results for treating digestive disorders. It helps when the digestive system is weak. It treats stomach problems and nausea. Sage improves memory loss, and improves the voice. Sage may be taken in capsules. **Sage may elevate blood pressure for some people when taken excessively.** Sage may be kept in the kitchen and used as a spice. If it is taken as a tea, use ¼ teaspoon of Sage herb powder to one cup of boiling water. Sage may be taken as often as you feel the need. For chronic digestive disorders it can be taken once or twice a day, for two to five days, or until desired results are reached. For some, once or twice a week can be beneficial.

Herbs for your blood type: Sage is highly beneficial for people with blood type B. It is neutral for people with blood type O, A, and AB.

Contains: sodium, sulphur, vitamins A, B complex, and C.

Uva Ursi

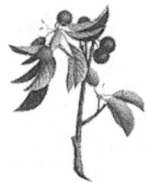

UVA URSI will assist with treating digestive disorders. It should be taken in combination with other digestive healing herbs. **Do not use Uva Ursi during pregnancy: it may cause damage to the fetus.** It increases the flow of urine and acts as a disinfectant to the system. Uva Ursi will turn the urine a dark green, do not panic, it is normal. Uva Ursi may be taken in capsules. If it is taken as a tea, use ¼ teaspoon of Uva Ursi to one cup of boiling water. Uva Ursi may be taken as often as you feel the need. For treating digestive disorders it may be taken once or twice a day, for two to five days, or until desired results are reached. For some, once or twice a week can be beneficial.

Contains: iron, manganese, trace minerals, and vitamin A.

DIGESTIVE DISORDERS

HERBS:

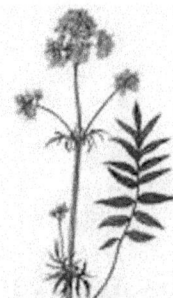

Valerian

VALERIAN can be helpful for treating digestive disorders. It is soothing and relaxing to the system. It treats gas and is best used in combination with other herbs. Use Valerian only for a short period to avoid mental depression. It helps to increase low concentration of blood sugar. **Do not give Valerian to children under age twelve.** Valerian should be taken at bedtime: it acts as a sedative when taken, but offers no drowsy after-effect. Valerian may be taken in capsules. If it is taken as a tea, use ¼ teaspoon of Valerian herb powder to one cup of boiling water. Valerian may be taken as often as you feel the need. For treating digestive disorders it may be taken once or twice a day, for two to three days, or until desired results are reached. For some, once or twice a week can be beneficial.

Herbs for your blood type: Valerian is highly beneficial for people with blood type A. It is neutral for people with blood type O, B and AB.

Contains: vitamins A and C, iron, sodium, potassium, niacin, calcium, magnesium, manganese, silicon, and selenium.

GALLSTONES

Barberry

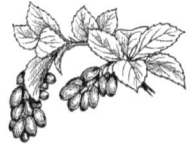

BARBERRY will assist with treating gallstones. It helps to eliminate them from the body. Barberry relieves the body of the effects of a sluggish gallbladder, and strengthens the entire system. **Do not take Barberry excessively it may cause depression.** It dilates blood vessels, which is good for high blood pressure. Barberry may be taken in capsules. If it is taken as a tea, use ¼ teaspoon of Barberry herb powder to one cup of boiling water. Barberry may be taken as often as you feel the need. For treating gallstones it may be taken once or twice a day, for two to seven days, or until desired results are reached. For some once or twice a week can be helpful.

Contains: iron, manganese, phosphorus, and vitamin C.

Black Cohosh

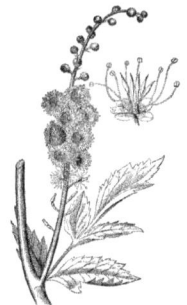

BLACK COHOSH will help to rid the body of gallstones. It gives great results for treating spinal meningitis, fevers, epilepsy, and tuberculosis. **Black Cohosh should be used in small amounts or it can cause a headache.** It lowers the heart rate slightly but increases the pulse rate. It reduces hot flashes, and can be taken as a sedative. **Black Cohosh will induce labor during pregnancy.** It may be taken in capsules. When

GALLSTONES

HERBS:

Black Cohosh is taken as a tea, use 1/8th teaspoon or less of Black Cohosh herb powder to one cup of boiling water. Black Cohosh may be taken as often as you feel the need. For treating gallstones it may be taken once or twice a day, for five to ten days, or until desired results are reached. For some, once or twice a week can give results in a short period.

Contains: calcium, potassium, iron, magnesium, manganese, niacin, phosphorus, selenium, silicon, sodium, sulphur, vitamins A, B1, B2, C, K, F, and zinc.

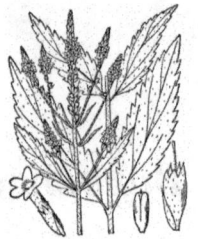

Blue Vervain

BLUE VERVAIN can assist with treating gallstones. It treats indigestion, insomnia, poor circulation, and lung congestion. It offers a calm and tranquilizing effect to the entire system. It is a soothing herb. A large amount of Blue Vervain taken at once may cause vomiting. It may be taken in capsules. If it is taken as a tea, use ¼ teaspoon of Blue Vervain herb powder to one cup of boiling water. Blue Vervain may be taken as often as you feel the need. For treating gallstones it may be taken once a day for five to ten days, until desired results are reached. For some, once or twice a week can be helpful for two to three weeks.

Contains: vitamin C, calcium, manganese, and vitamin E

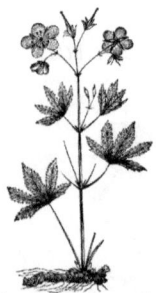

Buchu

BUCHU will aid with treating gallstones. It treats chronic kidney problems, and offers excellent results for prostate problems. Buchu will increase urination. It may be taken in capsules. If it is taken as a tea, use ¼ teaspoon of Buchu herb powder to one cup of boiling water. Buchu may be taken as often as you feel the need. For treating gallstones it may be taken once a day for two to five days, or until desired results are reached. For some, once or twice a week for two to three week can be helpful.

Contains bioflavonoids.

GALLSTONES

HERBS:

*Buckthorn

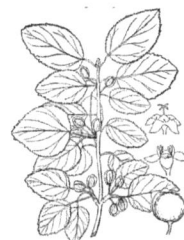

BUCKTHORN is excellent for treating chronic gallstones. It can be used to stimulate a sluggish gallbladder. Buckthorn treats cancer and chronic constipation. It will cause griping and cramps when used excessively. Buckthorn may be taken in capsules. If is taken as a tea, use ¼ teaspoon of Buckthorn herb powder to one cup of boiling water. Buckthorn may be taken as often as you feel the need. For chronic gallstones it may be taken once or twice a day for two to seven days, or until desired results are reached. For some, once or twice a week can be beneficial.

Contains vitamin C.

Burdock

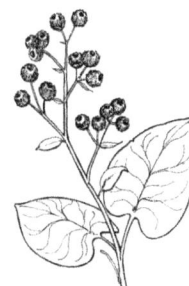

BURDOCK will help with riding the system of gallstones. It is a blood purifier that treats cancer, kidney, and liver problems. Burdock is excellent for treating gout, and it increases urine flow. **Burdock taken in an excessive amount at once may cause vomiting.** Burdock may be taken in capsules. If it is taken as a tea, use ¼ teaspoon of Burdock herb powder to one cup of boiling water. Burdock may be taken as often as you feel the need. For treating gallstones it may be taken once a day for three to five days, or until desired results are reached. For some, once or twice a a week can be helpful.

Herbs for your blood type: Burdock is highly beneficial for people with blood type A and AB. It is neutral for people with blood type B. People with blood type O should avoid this herb it will cause excessive blood thinning and excessive bleeding for them.

Contains: vitamins A, B complex, C, E, iron, zinc, and sulphur.

GALLSTONES

*Cascara Sagrada

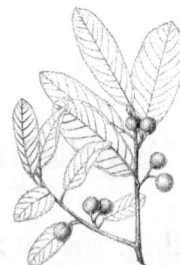

CASCARA SAGRADA will rid the system of gallstones. It treats a sluggish gallbladder. It is excellent for treating chronic constipation and liver disorders. Cascara Sagrada may be taken in capsules. If it is taken as a tea, use ¼ teaspoon of Cascara Sagrada herb powder to one cup of boiling water. Cascara Sagrada may be taken as often as you feel the need. For treating gallstones it may be taken once a day for two to five days, or until desired results are reached. For some, once or twice a week will be beneficial for desired results.

Contains: calcium, potassium, B complex, manganese, lead, aluminum, and tin.

Chamomile

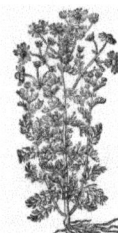

CHAMOMILE will assist with treating gallstones. It is soothing to the entire system, treating poor circulation, fevers, and drug addiction. Chamomile treats peptic ulcers, tumors, and insomnia. It will increase the appetite. Chamomile can be taken in capsules, if it is taken as a tea, use ¼ teaspoon of Chamomile herb powder to one cup of boiling water. Chamomile may be taken as often as you feel the need. For treating gallstones it may be taken once or twice a day, for two to seven days, or until desired results are reached.

Herbs for your blood type: Chamomile is highly beneficial for people with blood type A and AB. It is neutral for people with blood type O, and B.

Contains: potassium, calcium, iron, manganese, and vitamins A and zinc.

GALLSTONES

Chicory

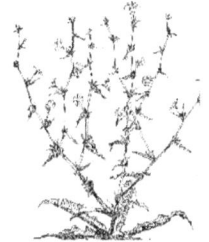

CHICORY can be helpful for treating gallstones. It is excellent for riding the system of calcium deposits. It purifies the blood and is excellent for treating liver disorders. It is a mild tonic, It may be taken in capsules. If it is taken as a tea, use ¼ teaspoon of Chicory herb powder to one cup of boiling water. Chicory may be taken as often as you feel the need. For gallstones it may be taken once or twice a day, for two to seven days, or until desired results are reached. For some, once or twice a week can be helpful.

Contains: a high amount of vitamins A, B, C, K, and P.

Dandelion

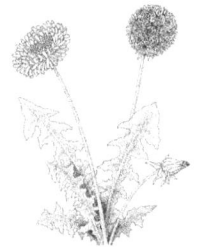

DANDELION will aid with the treatment of gallstones. It is excellent for treating gallbladder problems, hepatitis, jaundice, kidney infections, and liver disorders. **Dandelion may elevate blood pressure for some people when taken excessively.** Dandelion may be taken in capsules. If it is taken as a tea, use ¼ teaspoon of Dandelion herb powder to one cup of boiling water. Dandelion may be taken as often as you feel the need. For treating gallstones it may be taken once or twice a day, for two to ten days, or until desired results are reached. For some, once or twice a week can be beneficial.

   Herbs for your blood type: Dandelion is highly beneficial for people with blood type O. It is neutral for people with blood type A, B, and AB.

Contains: calcium, vitamin A, B, C, and E, sodium, potassium, iron, nickel, tin, copper, magnesium, manganese, sulphur, and zinc.

GALLSTONES

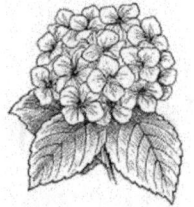

*Hydrangea

HYDRANGEA is an excellent herb to use for treating gallstones; it sends the stones through the bowels and bladder. It is excellent for bladder infection. **Hydrangea may elevate blood pressure for some people when it is taken excessively.** Hydrangea may be taken in capsules. When it is taken as a tea, use ¼ teaspoon of Hydrangea herb powder to one cup of boiling water. Hydrangea may be taken as often as you feel the need. For treating gallstones it may be taken once or twice a day, for two to ten days, or until desired results are reached.

Contains: sodium, sulphur, calcium, iron, potassium, and magnesium.

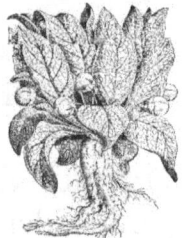

Mandrake

MANDRAKE can be helpful for treating gallstones; it is best used in combination with other herbs for treating gallstones, due to its toxicity. It can be irritating to the GI tract. It is great for removing tumors and treating chronic liver diseases. It will gripe the stomach when used in large amounts. **It is a laxative. Do not use Mandrake during pregnancy.** It may be taken in capsules. When it is taken as a tea use 1/8th teaspoon or less of Mandrake herb powder to two cups of boiling water. Mandrake may be taken as often as you feel the need. For gallstones it may be taken once or twice a week for two to three weeks for results.

Contents: vitamin information unknown.

GALLSTONES

Oatstraw

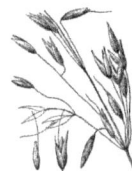

OATSTRAW can be helpful for treating gallstones. It helps with treating gallbladder problems, indigestion, and the bladder. It helps to treat the kidneys, liver, and nervous conditions. Oatstraw will help with recovery from an illness, or drug withdrawals. It helps to lower blood sugar levels, blood pressure and cholesterol. Oatstraw stimulates the appetite. It should be taken at bedtime. Oatstraw may be taken in capsules. If it is taken as a tea, use ½ teaspoon of Oatstraw herb powder to one cup of boiling water. Oatstraw may be taken as often as you feel the need. For treating gallstones it may be taken once or twice a day, for two to ten days, or until desired results are reached.

Contains: vitamins A, B1, B2, and E, and is high in calcium, and silicon.

*Parsley

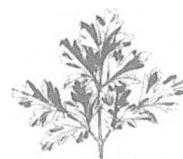

PARSLEY is excellent for treating chronic gallstones. It treats kidney stones, prostate glands, and gallbladder disorder. It helps with cancer prevention. It should be used in moderation during pregnancy: it will induce labor pains. After birth it will dry up mother's milk during the weaning period. Parsley may be taken in capsules, when it is taken as a tea, use ¼ teaspoons of Parsley herb powder to one cup of boiling water. Parsley may be taken as often as you feel the need.

Herbs for your blood type: Parsley is highly beneficial for people with blood type O and B. It is neutral for people with blood type A and AB.

Contains: vitamins A, B, and C, chlorophyll, iron, potassium, calcium, cobalt, copper, riboflavin, silicon sodium, sulphur, and thiamine.

GALLSTONES

HERBS:

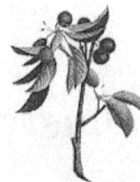

Uva Ursi

Uva Ursi will help to rid the body of gallstones. It treats bladder infections, digestive disorders, kidney infections, weak prostate glands, and chronic urethritis problems. Use a small amount in the beginning and increase the amount as necessary. **Do not use this herb during pregnancy: it could possibly be harmful to the fetus.** Uva Ursi increases the flow of urine and acts as a disinfectant. Uva Ursi will turn the urine a dark green do not panic it is normal. Uva Ursi may be taken in capsules. If it is taken as a tea, use ¼ teaspoon of Uva Ursi herb powder to one cup of boiling water. Uva Ursi may be taken as often as you feel the need. For treating the gallstones, it may be taken once or twice a day for two to ten days, or until desired results are reached. For some, once or twice a week can be beneficial.

Contains: iron, manganese, trace minerals, and vitamin A.

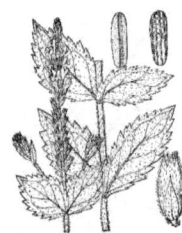

Vervain

Vervain can be a soothing herb for treating gallstones. It treats sluggish digestion problems, liver, and urinary problems. It is best known for treating nervous disorders, and will be helpful with treating insomnia. Vervain may be taken in capsules, if it is taken as a tea, use ¼ teaspoon of Vervain herb powder to one cup of boiling water. Vervain may be taken as often as you feel the need for treating gallstones it may be taken once or twice a day for two to ten days, or until desired results are reached. For some, once or twice a week can be helpful.

Contains: calcium, manganese, and vitamins C and E.

GALLSTONES

White Oak Bark

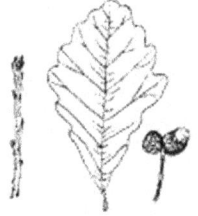

WHITE OAK BARK can be useful for treating gallstones. It treats gastrointestinal problems, bladder disorders, liver, and varicose veins. It treats PMS and it can be useful for treating external and internal bleeding. **White Oak Bark may elevate blood pressure for some people when taken excessively.** White Oak Bark may be taken in capsules. If it is taken as a tea, use ¼ teaspoon of White Oak Bark herb powder to one cup of boiling water. White oak Bark may be taken as often as you feel the need. For treating gallstones it may be taken once or twice a day, for two to ten days, or until desired results are reached.

Contains: sodium, cobalt, lead, iodine, potassium, calcium, sulphur, and vitamin B12.

GLANDS

*Bayberry

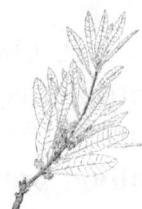

BAYBERRY is excellent for treating the glands. It soothes and relieves painful and infected glands. It is helpful with colds, chills, and sore throats. It can be used as a gargle for tonsillitis and offers vitality to the body. It may be taken in capsules. If it is taken as a tea, use ¼ teaspoon of Bayberry herb powder to one cup of boiling water. Bayberry may be taken as often as you feel the need. For gland problems it may be taken once or twice a day, for two to seven days, or until desired results are reached. For some, once or twice a week can be beneficial.

Contains: potassium, sodium, niacin, calcium, magnesium, manganese, silicon, zinc, vitamins B1, B2, and C.

Buchu

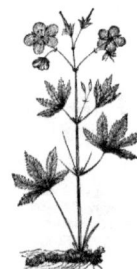

BUCHU can be helpful with treating the glands. It soothes lower back pains and treats painful urinary problems. It treats a weak bladder and kidney problems. It will assist with lowering blood pressure. Urination increases while using Buchu. Buchu should be used in combination with other herbs, such as Squaw Vine. Buchu may be taken in capsules. If it is taken as a tea, use ¼ teaspoon of Buchu herb powder to one cup of boiling water. Buchu may be taken as often as you feel the need. For treating the glands it may be taken once or twice a day for two to five days, or until desired results are reached. For some, once or twice a week can be helpful.

Contains bioflavonoids.

GLANDS

HERBS:

Chicory

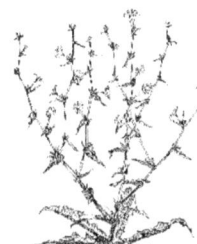

CHICORY will assist with treating the glands. It treats inflammation, jaundice, calcium deposits, and the spleen. It helps with treating stiff joints and gout. Chicory is a blood purifier. It may be taken in capsules. If it is taken as a tea, use ¼ teaspoon of Chicory herb powder to one cup of boiling water. Chicory may be taken as often as you feel the need. For treating the glands it may be taken once or twice a day, for two to five days, or until desired results are reached. For some two or three times a week will give relief.

Contains: a high amount of vitamins A, B, C, K, and P.

*Echinacea

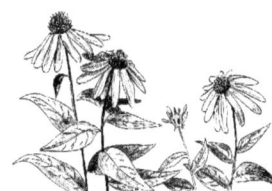

ECHINACEA is excellent for treating the glands. It treats the lymph glands, prostate glands, tonsillitis, bladder infection, and syphilis. Echinacea is an antibiotic that cleans the blood. Echinacea increases white blood cells. Echinacea may be taken in capsules. If it is taken as tea, use ¼ teaspoon of Echinacea herb powder to one cup of boiling water. Echinacea may be taken as often as you feel the need. For treating the glands it may be taken once or twice a day, for two to five days, or until desired results are reached. For some, two or three times a week can be beneficial.

Herbs for your blood type: Echinacea is highly beneficial for people with blood type A and AB. It is neutral for people with blood type B. People with blood type O should avoid this herb. Echinacea will cause excessive blood thinning for people with blood type O.

Contains: vitamins A, C, E, iron, iodine, copper, sulphur, and potassium

GLANDS

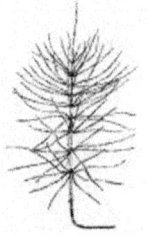

*Horsetail

HORSETAIL can be an excellent herb for treating the glands. It treats glandular disorders, bladder problems, kidney stones, and circulation problems. It treats parasites and urinary ulcers. Horsetail is a diuretic and will increase urination. **Horsetail may elevate blood pressure for some people when taken excessively at once.** Horsetail may be taken in capsules. If it is taken as a tea, use ¼ teaspoon of Horsetail herb powder to one cup of boiling water. Horsetail may be taken as often as you feel the need. For chronic glandular disorders it may be taken two or three times a day, for two to seven days, or until desired results are reached. For some, two or three times a week will be beneficial.

Contains: sodium, iron, iodine, copper, vitamin E, and has a high content of silicon and selenium.

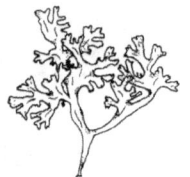

*Irish Moss

IRISH MOSS can be terrific for treating the glands. It treats bladder problems, radiation poisoning, and reduces the appetite. Iris Moss is high in iodine and treats thyroid problems. It may be taken in capsules, if it is taken as a tea, use ¼ teaspoon of Irish Moss herb powder to one cup of boiling water. Irish Moss may be taken as often as you feel the need. For treating chronic gland problems it may be taken once or twice a day, for two to seven days, or until desired results are reached. For some two or three times a week will give relief.

Contains: a high amount of vitamins A, B, C, K, and P.

GLANDS

HERBS:

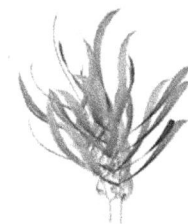

*Kelp

KELP can be excellent for treating enlarged glands. It balances overactive or under active thyroid glands, treats infections, radiation poisoning, and obesity. Kelp treats cancer growths, fingernails, and offers energy to the entire system. Kelp helps the brain to function normally. Kelp may be taken in capsules. If it is taken as a tea, use ¼ teaspoon of Kelp herb powder to one cup of boiling water. Kelp may be taken as often as you feel the need. For treating enlarged glands it may be taken once or twice a day, for two to seven days, or until desired results are reached. For some, once or twice a week will be beneficial for the glands.

Contains: calcium, chlorine, sulphur, silicon, zinc, manganese, aluminum, potassium, copper, nickel, iron, silver, phosphorus, vanadium, B complex, vitamins A, C, E, and K, and has a very high content of iodine and minerals.

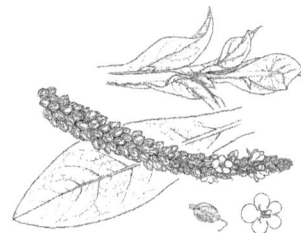

*Mullein

MULLEIN can be fantastic for treating swollen glands. It treats swollen membranes, inflammation, and pain. It is excellent for treating swollen joints and respiratory problems. It's great for stemming bleeding in the bowels, and the lungs. Mullein is best taken at bedtime because it will cause sleepiness. It may be taken in capsules. If it is taken as a tea, use ¼ teaspoon of Mullein herb powder to one cup of boiling water. Mullein may be taken as often as you feel the need. For treating swollen glands it may be taken once or twice a day, for two to five days, or until desired results are reached. For some, once or twice a week will be beneficial.

Herbs for your blood type: Mullein is neutral for people with blood type O, and A. People with Blood type B and AB should avoid this herb.

Contains: magnesium, potassium, and sulphur. Mullein is very high in iron.

GLANDS

HERBS:

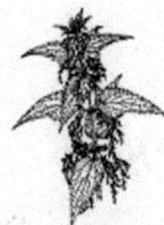

*Saw Palmetto

SAW PALMETTO can be highly beneficial for treating the glands. It treats the sexual glands and organs. It affects all of the glandular tissues. It relieves membrane irritation in the throat, and has been known to increase breast size. It regulates hormones, and treats enlarged prostate glands. Saw Palmetto is a sexual stimulant. It is great for men that suffer from impotence due to alcohol disease. It may be taken in capsules. If it is taken as a tea use ½ teaspoon of Saw Palmetto herb powder to one cup of boiling water. Saw Palmetto may be taken as often as you feel the need. For treating chronic gland problems it may be taken once or twice a day, for two to seven days, or until desired results are reached. For some, two or three times a week can be beneficial.

Contains vitamin A.

GOUT

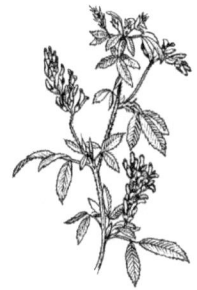

*Alfalfa

ALFALFA can be very beneficial for treating gout. It treats swelling, inflammation in the joints, and minor pain. It removes deposits and fibrosis of the inner arteries. Alfalfa helps to prevent colon cancer when taken over an extended period. It will enhance the immune system and treat acidity. Alfalfa may be taken in capsules. If it is taken as a tea, use ¼ teaspoon of Alfalfa herb powder to one cup of boiling water. Alfalfa may be taken as often as you feel the need. For chronic painful gout it may be taken two or three times a day for two to seven days, or until the desired results are reached. For some two or three times a week will help with prevention.

Herbs for your blood type: Alfalfa is highly beneficial for people with blood type A. It is neutral for people with blood type B and AB. People with blood type O should avoid this herb it will cause excessive blood thinning for them.

Contains: vitamins A, B complex, D, E, and K, iron, potassium, magnesium, protein, sodium, sulfur, and phosphorus, and is very high in calcium, chlorophyll, and vitamin B12.

GOUT

HERBS:

Angelica

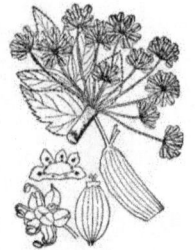

ANGELICA will assist with treating gout. It treats inflammation, rheumatism, arthritis, and helps to lower blood pressure. Angelica will stimulate the appetite, and increase urination. Angelica should be used with caution if you are a diabetic: it will elevate blood sugar levels. Do not take Angelica if you suffer excessive bleeding. **Angelica should not be used during pregnancy it may cause a miscarriage.** Angelica may be taken in capsules. If it is taken as a tea, use ¼ teaspoon of Angelica herb powder to one cup of boiling water. Angelica may be taken as often as you feel the need. For treating painful gout it may be taken two or three times a day for two to seven days, or until the desired results are reached. For some two or three times a week can be helpful.

Contains: vitamins E, B 12, and calcium.

Birch

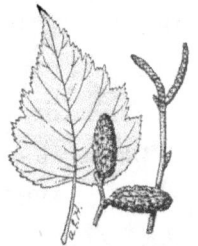

BIRCH will assist with treating gout. It treats pain, arthritis, rheumatism, and cancer. It is a healing herb and acts very similar to aspirin. Birch is a diuretic and a sedative; it may be taken at bedtime for insomnia. It may be taken in capsules. If it is taken as a tea, use ¼ teaspoon of Birch herb powder to one cup of boiling water. Birch may be taken as often as you feel the need. For treating painful gout it may be taken two or three times a day for two to five days, or until the desired results are reached. For some, two or three times a week will help with prevention.

Contains: copper, sodium, calcium, iron, magnesium, potassium, silicon, vitamin A, B1, B2, C, and E.

GOUT

Buckthorn

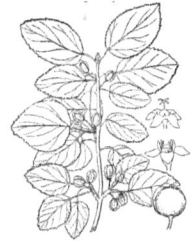

BUCKTHORN can be of assistance in treating gout. It treats rheumatism, cancer, parasites, warts, and chronic constipation. Buckthorn will cause griping and cramps when it is taken excessively. It removes lead poisoning from the body and treats liver problems. Buckthorn may be taken in capsules. If it is taken as a tea, use ¼ teaspoon of Buckthorn herb powder to one cup of boiling water. Buckthorn may be taken as often as you feel the need. For treating gout it may be taken two or three times a day for two to five days, or until the desired results are reached. For some two or three times a week will offer prevention.

Contains vitamin C.

*Burdock

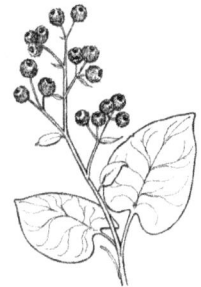

BURDOCK can be excellent to use for treating gout. It treats arthritis, bursitis, rheumatism, inflammation, sciatica, swelling, and cancer. Urine will increase while taking Burdock. BURDOCK MAY CAUSE VOMITING WHEN TAKEN EXCESSIVELY AT ONCE. It may be taken in capsules. If it is taken as a tea, use ¼ teaspoon of Burdock herb powder to one cup of boiling water. Burdock may be taken as often as you feel the need. For chronic painful gout it may be taken two or three times a day for two to five days, or until the desired results are reached. For some two or three times a week can be beneficial.

Herbs for your blood type: Burdock is highly beneficial for people with blood type A and AB. It is neutral for people with blood type B. People with blood type O should avoid this herb it will cause excessive blood thinning and excessive bleeding for them."

Contains: vitamins A, B complex, C, E, iron, zinc, and sulphur.

GOUT

HERBS:

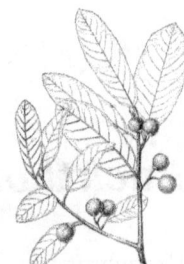

Cascara Sagrada

CASCARA SAGRADA will help to relieve gout. It treats congestion, lowers blood pressure, and treats chronic and toxic bowel syndrome. It treats Jaundice, parasites, worms, and stomach disorders. Cascara Sagrada may be taken in capsules. If it is taken as a tea, use ¼ teaspoon of Cascara Sagrada herb powder to one cup of boiling water. Cascara Sagrada may be taken as often as you feel the need. For treating gout it may be taken once or twice a day, for two to five days, or until the desired results are reached. For some two or three times a week will help with prevention.

Contains: calcium, potassium, B complex, manganese, lead, aluminum, and tin.

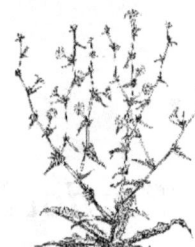

Chicory

CHICORY will assist with treating gout. It treats arthritis and inflammation. It removes calcium deposits and fibrosis of the inner arteries. Chicory is a blood purifier that treats jaundice and liver problems. It may be taken in capsules. If it is taken as a tea, use ¼ teaspoon of Chicory herb powder to one cup of boiling water. Chicory may be taken as often as you feel the need. For treating gout it may be taken two or three times a day for two to five days, or until the desired results are reached. For some once or twice a week will help with prevention.

Contains: a high amount of vitamins A, B, C, K, and P.

GOUT

Comfrey

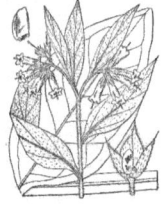

COMFREY will offer assistance with treating gout. It treats swelling, bursitis, rheumatism, and fractures. It will also be helpful with treating gangrene infections, leg cramps, and sprains. Comfrey may be taken in capsules, if it is taken as a tea use ¼ teaspoon of Comfrey herb powder to one cup of boiling water. Comfrey may be taken as often as you feel the need. For treating gout it may be taken two or three times a day for two to five days, or until the desired results are reached. For some two or three days a week will be helpful for prevention.

Contains: vitamins A, C, iron, sulphur, copper, zinc, magnesium. Comfrey is very high in calcium, potassium, and protein.

Couch Grass

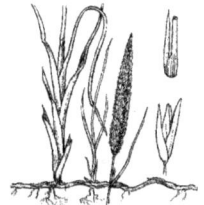

COUCH GRASS can be beneficial for treating gout. It also treats rheumatism, bladder infections, fevers, jaundice, syphilis, and urinary infections. It may be taken in capsules. If it is taken as a tea, use ¼ teaspoon of Couch Grass herb powder to one cup of boiling water. Couch Grass may be taken as often as you feel the need. For treating gout it may be taken two or three times a day for two to five days, or until the desired results are reached. For some once or twice a week will help with prevention.

Contains: sodium, potassium, calcium, and magnesium. Couch Grass is high in silicon, vitamin A, C, and B complex.

GOUT

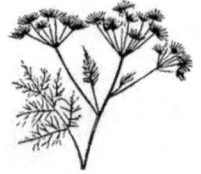

Fennel

FENNEL will help to treat gout. It lowers cholesterol, suppresses the appetite, and treats obesity. Fennel treats uric acid and water retention. It expels gas and treats acid in the stomach. It also treats nausea and indigestion problems. Fennel will suppress the appetite. **Fennel may increase the blood pressure for some people when taken excessively at once.** Fennel can be used as a spice. It may be taken in capsules. If it is taken as a tea, use ¼ teaspoon of Fennel herb powder to one cup of boiling water. Fennel may be taken as often as you feel the need. For treating gout it may be taken two or three times a day, for two to seven days, or until desired results are reached. For some two or three times a week will be helpful.

Contains: sodium, potassium, sulphur, and is high in vitamin A.

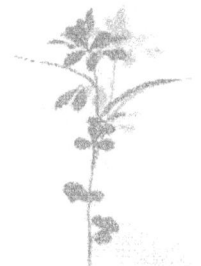

Fenugreek

FENUGREEK can offer success with treating gout. It is also excellent for dissolving cholesterol, it treats allergies, and lymphatic cancer. It is great for treating emphysema and hay fever. Women who wish to get pregnant should not use fenugreek it will impede the progress. Fenugreek may be taken in capsules. If it is taken as a tea, use ¼ teaspoon of Fenugreek herb powder to one cup of boiling water. Fenugreek may be taken as often as you feel the need. For treating gout it may be taken two or three times a day for two to five days, or until the desired results are reached. For some two or three times a week will assist with prevention.

Herbs for your blood type: Fenugreek is highly beneficial for people with blood type O, and A. People with blood type B, or AB should avoid this herb.

Contains: vitamins B1, B2, iron, and choline. Fenugreek is very high in vitamins A and D.

GOUT

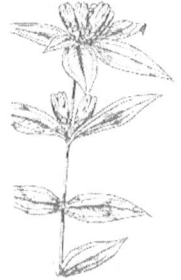

Gentian

GENTIAN can be helpful with treating gout. It also treats circulation, anal itch, and it strengthens the digestive system. Gentian stimulates the appetite, and treats hysteria. Buckthorn or Kelp should be taken in combination with this herb. Gentian may be taken in capsules, if it is taken as a tea, use ¼ teaspoon of Gentian herb powder to one cup of boiling water. Gentian may be taken as often as you feel the need. For treating gout it may be taken two or three times a day for two to five days, or until the desired results are reached. For some two or three times a week will help with prevention.

Contains: sulphur, tin, lead, manganese, zinc, niacin, and is high in iron.

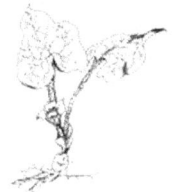

Ginger

GINGER will assist with treating gout. It also treats poor circulation, cramps, paralysis, toothache, and vomiting. Do not take aspirin while using Ginger; it will inhibit the performance of Ginger. Ginger is best found in the produce section of the grocery market. It may be taken in capsules. If it is taken as a tea, grate the ginger and steep it in a container with a covered lid. Ginger may be taken as often as you feel the need. For gout it may be taken two or three times a day for two to seven days, or until the desired results are reached. For some, two or three times a week will help with prevention.

Herbs for your blood type: Ginger is highly beneficial for people with blood type O, A, B, and AB.

Contains: vitamins A, B complex, C, calcium, iron, sodium, potassium, and magnesium.

GOUT

HERBS:

Horseradish

HORSERADISH will help to ease the pain of gout. It treats rheumatism, water retention, and wounds. It may be taken in capsules. If it is taken as a tea, use ¼ teaspoon of Horseradish herb powder to one cup of boiling water. Horseradish may be taken as often as you feel the need. For treating gout it may be taken once or twice a day for two to seven days, or until desires results are reached. For some, once or twice a week can be helpful.

Contains: vitamins A, B complex, iron, calcium, sodium, and phosphorus.

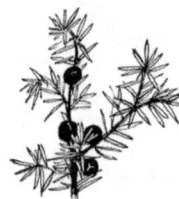

Juniper

JUNIPER will offer assistance in treating gout. It treats rheumatism, bladder problems, and excessive bleeding. It is also excellent for treating urinary problems and water retention. **Juniper is not recommended for pregnant women.** It produces natural insulin in the body. It can be used as a poultice for boils. Juniper may be taken in capsules. If it is taken as a tea, use ¼ teaspoon of Juniper herb powder to one cup of boiling water. Juniper may be taken as often as you feel the need. For treating gout it may be taken once or twice a day, for two to seven days, or until desired results are reached. For some once or twice a week can be helpful for prevention.

Contains: a high amount of vitamin C, aluminum, sulphur, and copper.

GOUT

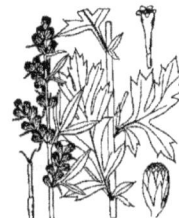

*Mugwort

Mugwort can be helpful for treating gout. It treats poor circulation, rheumatism, lumbago, and obesity. It is best used externally as a liniment. Mugwort should not be used in large amounts; it can be toxic and should only be used for short periods of time. Do not use it excessively. **Mugwort is not recommended for children at all. This herb will aide in the promotion of menstruation and should not be used by pregnant women.** Mugwort should not be used more than once in a week. Mugwort may be taken in capsules. If it is taken as a tea, use 1/8th teaspoon or less of Mugwort herb powder to one cup of boiling water.

Content: vitamin information unknown.

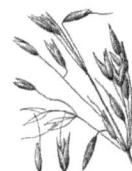

Oatstraw

Oatstraw will help with the relief of gout; it treats rheumatism, arthritis, brittle bones, shingles, and the urinary system. It helps to lower blood pressure and cholesterol. Oatstraw will help with recovery from an illness, or drug withdrawals. It can be helpful for treating thyroid and estrogen deficiency. Oatstraw stimulates the appetite. It should be taken at bedtime. Oatstraw may be taken in capsules. If it is taken as a tea, use ¼ teaspoon of Oatstraw herb powder to one cup of boiling water. Oatstraw may be taken as often as you feel the need. For treating gout it may be taken two or three times a day for two to five days, or until the desired results are reached. For some once or twice a week can help with prevention.

Contains: vitamins A, B1, B2, and E, and is high in calcium and silicon.

GOUT

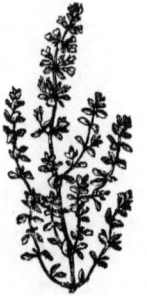

Pennyroyal

PENNYROYAL can be very effective for treating gout. It treats cramps, fainting, pleurisy, toothaches, and tuberculosis. Pennyroyal is very soothing and will promote perspiration and menstruation. **Do not use Pennyroyal during pregnancy it has been known to induce spontaneous abortion.** Kelp should be used in combination with Pennyroyal. It imay be taken in capsules. If it is taken as a tea, use ¼ teaspoon of Pennyroyal herb powder to one cup of boiling water. Pennyroyal may be taken as often as you feel the need. For treating gout it may be taken two or three times a day for two to five days, or until the desired results are reached. For some, once or twice a week can be effective.

Contains: sodium and lead.

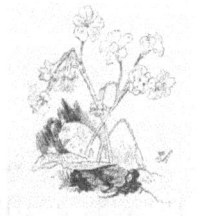

*Queen of The Meadow

QUEEN OF THE MEADOW is excellent for treating gout. It treats bursitis, gravel, rheumatism, and urinary problems. It may be taken in capsules. If it is taken as a tea, use ¼ teaspoon of Queen of The Meadow herb powder to one cup of boiling water. Queen of The Meadow may be taken as often as you feel the need. For treating chronic gout it may be taken two or three times a day, for two to five days, or until desired results are reached. For some, once or twice a week can be effective.

Contains: vitamins A, C, and D.

GOUT

HERBS:

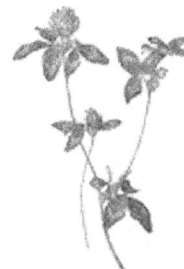

Red Clover

RED CLOVER can be helpful with treating gout. It treats rheumatism, leukemia, and strengthens the ovaries. It treats cancer, and rectal irritation. Red Clover may be taken in capsules. If it is taken as a tea, use ¼ teaspoon of Red Clover herb powder to one cup of boiling water. Red Clover may be taken as often as you feel the need. For treating gout it may be taken once or twice a day, for two to five days, or until the desired results are reached. For some, once or twice a week can be helpful for prevention.

Contains: vitamins A, B complex, calcium, sodium, nickel, manganese, tin, and is high in iron and calcium.

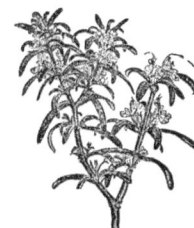

Rosemary

ROSEMARY can be helpful for treating gout. It improves circulation, treats rheumatism, inflammation in the joints, prostate and muscle spasms. Rosemary promotes hair growth. When Rosemary is used with Myrrh it will stop bleeding gums. It may be taken in capsules. If it is taken as a tea, use ¼ teaspoon of Rosemary herb powder to one cup of boiling water. Rosemary may be taken as often as you feel the need. For treating gout it may be taken once or twice a day, for two to seven days, or until desired results are reached. For some, once or twice a week can be helpful.

Contains: iron, sodium, potassium, zinc, phosphorus, magnesium, vitamins A and C, and is high in calcium.

GOUT

HERBS:

*Safflower

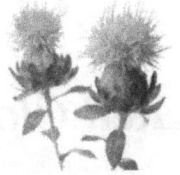

SAFFLOWER can be very beneficial for treating chronic gout. It will increase perspiration, and increase the flow of urine. Safflower stimulates the pancreas, clears phlegm from the lungs, and will produce temporary insulin. It may be taken in capsules. If it is taken as a tea use 1/8th teaspoon of safflower herb powder to one cup of boiling water. Safflower may be taken as often as you feel the need. For chronic gout it may be taken two or three times a day for two to seven days, or until desired results are reached. For some, once or twice a week will offer relief.

Contains vitamin K.

*Saffron

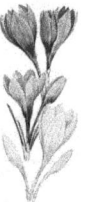

SAFFRON can be great for treating gout. It treats rheumatism and poor circulation, it offers energy to the system. It can be helpful with treating cancer and headaches. It can be great for liver and urinary problems. It may be taken in capsules. If it is taken as a tea, use ¼ teaspoon of Saffron herb powder to one cup of boiling water. Saffron may be taken as often as you feel the need. For treating chronic gout it may be taken two or three times a day, for two to seven days, or until desired results are reached. For some, once or twice a day will offer relief.

Contains: sodium, calcium, potassium, and vitamins A and B 12.

GOUT

HERBS:

*Sarsaparilla

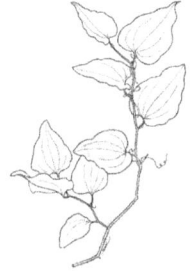

Sarsaparilla is excellent for treating gout. It treats achy joints, and chronic rheumatism. It purifies the blood, treats sexual, and urinary problems. Some people use it as a natural steroid because it builds muscles. Sarsaparilla may be taken in capsules. If it is taken as a tea, use ¼ teaspoon of Sarsaparilla herb powder to one cup of boiling water. Sarsaparilla may be taken as often as you feel the need. For chronic gout it may be taken two or three times a day for two to five days, or until the desired results are reached. For some, once or twice a week will offer relief.

Herbs for your blood type: Sarsaparilla is highly beneficial for people with blood type O. It is neutral for people with blood type A, B and AB.

Contains: iron, sodium, silicon, sulphur, zinc, iodine, copper, manganese, vitamins A, B complex, C, and D.

*Thyme

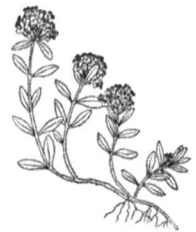

Thyme can be an excellent choice for treating gout. It treats rheumatism, sciatica, and migraine headaches. Thyme may be kept in the kitchen and used as a spice. **Thyme may elevate blood pressure for some people when taken excessively at once.** Thyme may be taken in capsules. If it is taken as a tea, use ¼ teaspoon of Thyme herb powder to one cup of boiling water. Thyme may be taken as often as you feel the need. For chronic gout it may be taken two or three times a day for two to three days, or until the desired results are reached. For some, once or twice a week will offer relief.

Herbs for your blood type: Thyme is highly beneficial for people with blood type O and B. It is neutral for people with blood type A and AB.

Contains: sodium, iodine, sulphur, and vitamins C and D.

GOUT

Willow

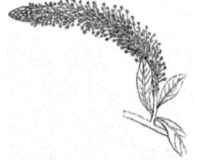

WILLOW will assist with treating gout. It treats rheumatism, inflammation in the joints, and ulcerations. Willow may be taken in capsules. If it is taken as a tea, use ¼ teaspoon of Willow herb powder to one cup of boiling water. Willow may be taken as often as you feel the need. For treating gout it may be taken once or twice a day, for two to five days, or until the desired results are reached. For some, once or twice a week will offer relief.

Herbs for your blood type: Willow is neutral for people with blood type O and A. People with Blood type B and AB should avoid this herb.

Contains: magnesium, potassium, and sulphur, and is very high in iron.

HEART

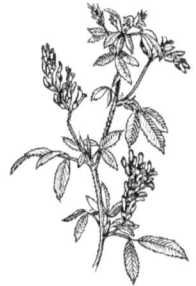

Alfalfa

ALFALFA will help to treat a diseased heart. It purifies the blood, treats chronic weakness, insomnia, and it stimulates the appetite. Alfalfa wards off infections, stimulates the pituitary gland, and treats acidity. Alfalfa may be taken in capsules. If it is taken as a tea, use ¼ teaspoon of Alfalfa herb powder to one cup of boiling water. Alfalfa may be taken as often as you feel the need. For diseased heart it may be taken two or three times a day for two to ten days, or until the desired results are reached. For some, two or three times a week will be beneficial.

Herbs for your blood type: Alfalfa is highly beneficial for people with blood type A. It is neutral for people with blood type B and AB. People with blood type O should avoid this herb it will cause excessive blood thinning for them.

Contains: vitamins A, B complex, D, E, and K, iron, potassium, magnesium, protein, sodium, sulfur, and phosphorus. Alfalfa is very high in calcium, chlorophyll, and vitamin B12.

HEART

Aloe

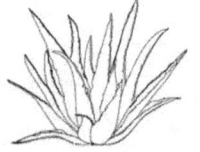

ALOE will increase oxygen flowing to the heart. It treats heartburn, psoriasis, and scar tissue. It treats allergies and it acts as a buffer for the HIV virus. Aloe may be taken in capsules. If it is taken as a tea, use ¼ teaspoon of Aloe herb powder to one cup of boiling water. Aloe may be taken as often as you feel the need. For treating the heart it may be taken two or three times a day for two to seven days, or until the desired results are reached. For some, two or three times a week will be beneficial.

Herbs for your blood type: Aloe is highly beneficial for people with blood type A. People with blood type O, B and AB should avoid using this herb as much as possible, internally. Externally, it is great for all blood types.

Contains: potassium, sodium, manganese, iron, and zinc.

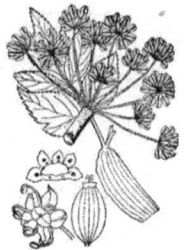

Angelica

ANGELICA will strengthen the heart; it lower blood pressure, and treat exhaustion, rheumatism, and toothaches. Angelica will stimulate the appetite, and increase urination. **Angelica should be used with caution if you are a diabetic; it will elevate blood sugar levels. Do not take Angelica if you suffer from excessive bleeding. Pregnant women should not use this herb during pregnancy: it may cause miscarriage.** Angelica may be taken in capsules. If it is taken as a tea, use ¼ teaspoon of Angelica herb powder to one cup of boiling water. Angelica may be taken as often as you feel the need. For heart disease it may be taken once or twice a day, for five to seven days, or until the desired results are reached. For some, two or three times a week will be beneficial.

Contains vitamins E, B 12, and calcium.

HEART

Astragalus

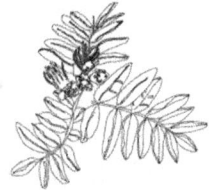

ASTRAGALUS can be very effective for treating a diseased heart. It treats edema, hypertension, stress, and muscle spasms. Astragalus increases white T-cells, and stimulates the immune system. Astragalus increases urination, it is a diuretic. It treats a prolapsed organ, and uterine cancer. It may be taken in capsules. If it is taken as a tea, use ¼ teaspoons of Astragalus herb powder to one cup of boiling water. Astragalus may be taken as often as you feel the need. For a diseased heart it may be taken once or twice a day, for two to seven days, or until the desired results are reached. For some, two or three times a week will be beneficial.

Contains: choline, betaine, and glucoronic acid.

Barberry

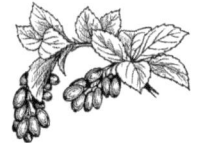

BARBERRY will assist with treating the heart. It treats heartburn, hypertension, indigestion, and arthritis. It can be effective for treating a variety of viruses, and stimulating the immune system. Barberry may be taken in capsules. When it is taken as a tea, use 1/8th teaspoon or less of Barberry herb powder to one cup of boiling water. Barberry may be taken as often as you feel the need. For the heart it may be taken once or twice a day, for three to five days, or until desired results are reached. For some, two or three times a week can be helpful.

Contains: iron, manganese, phosphorus, and vitamin C.

HEART

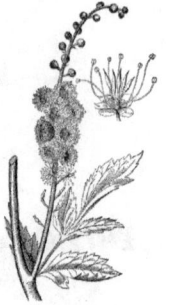

Black Cohosh

BLACK COHOSH can be effective for treating palpitations in the heart. It lowers the heart rate slightly, but increases the pulse rate. It treats inflammation, liver, and lumbago. Black Cohosh should be used in small amounts or it can cause a headache. It reduces hot flashes and is a sedative. **Black Cohosh will induce labor when pregnant.** Black Cohosh should be used in combination with other herbs. **Black Cohosh should be used in small amounts; it can cause a headache when taken excessively.** It may be taken in capsules.When it is taken as a tea, use 1/8th teaspoon or less of Black Cohosh herb powder, to one cup of boiling water. Black Cohosh may be taken as often as you feel the need. For heart palpitation it may be taken once or twice a day, for three to five days, or until desired results are reached. For some, two or three times a week can be helpful.

Contains: calcium, potassium, iron, magnesium, manganese, niacin, phosphorus, selenium, silicon, sodium, sulphur, vitamins A, B1, B2, C, K, and F, and zinc.

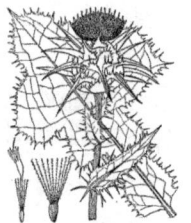

*Blessed Thistle

BLESSED THISTLE will strengthen the heart muscles. It strengthens the lungs, cancer, and increases blood circulation throughout the system. It brings oxygen to the brain. It may be taken in capsules. If it is taken as a tea, use ¼ teaspoon of Blessed Thistle herb powder to one cup of boiling water. Blessed Thistle may be taken as often as you feel the need. For chronic heart problems it may be taken two or three times a day, for five to seven days, or until desired results are reached. For some, once or twice a week will be beneficial.

Contains: B complex, calcium, iron, manganese, and potassium.

HEART

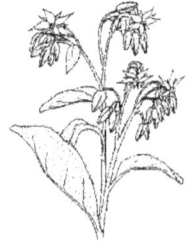

*Borage

BORAGE is great for strengthening the heart. It acts as a tonic for the heart, and treats phlegm and congestion in the lungs. Borage is great for treating inflammation of the eyes. Borage may be taken in capsules. If it is taken as a tea, use ¼ teaspoon of Borage herb powder to one cup of boiling water. Borage may be taken as often as you feel the need. For chronic heart problems it may be taken two or three times a day, for three to five days, or until desired results are reached. For some, once or twice a week will be beneficial.

Contains: calcium and potassium.

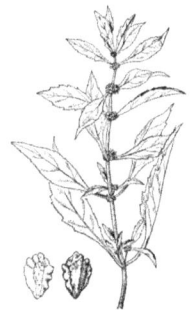

*Bugleweed

BUGLEWEED can be great for the heart. It is a tonic that treats rapid and irregular heartbeats. It treats edema. Bugleweed will lower the pulse. It may be taken in capsules. If it is taken as a tea, use ¼ teaspoon of Bugleweed herb powder to one cup of boiling water. Bugleweed may be taken as often as you feel the need. For chronic heart problems it may be taken once or twice a day, for two to seven days, or until the desired results are reached. For some, two or three times a week can be beneficial.

Contents: vitamin information unknown.

HEART

HERBS:

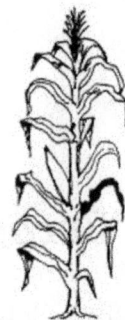

*Cornsilk

CORNSILK will help to strengthen a weak heart. It treats dropsy, edema, and urinary problems. Cornsilk is a diuretic. It may be taken in capsules, if it is taken as a tea use 1/8th teaspoon or less of Cornsilk herb powder to one cup of boiling water. Cornsilk may be taken as often as you feel the need. For chronic heart problems it may be taken once or twice a day, for three to seven days, or until desired results are reached. For some, once or twice a week can be beneficial.

Contains: vitamin B, silicon, and is very high in vitamin K.

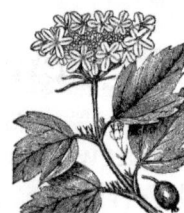

*Cramp Bark

CRAMP BARK is a tonic that treats the heart. It treats heart muscles, heart spasms, heart palpitations, and hypertension. Cramp Bark treats uterine cramps. It may be taken in capsules. If it is taken as a tea, use ¼ teaspoon of Cramp Bark herb powder to one cup of boiling water. Cramp Bark may be taken as often as you feel the need. For chronic heart problems it may be taken once or twice a day, for three to seven days, or until the desired results are reached. For some, once or twice a week can be beneficial.

Contains: calcium, potassium, magnesium, and is very high in vitamins C and K.

HEART

HERBS:

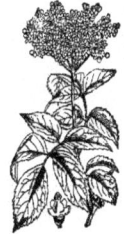

Dong Quai

DONG QUAI can help to strengthen the heart. It treats anemia, poor circulation, and helps to open blood vessels and treats nervousness. Dong Quai may be taken in capsules. If it is taken as a tea, use ¼ teaspoon of Dong Quai herb powder to one cup of boiling water. Dong Quai may be taken as often as you feel the need. For heart problems it may be taken once or twice a day, for three to five days, or until the desired results are reached. For some, once or twice a week can be helpful.

Herbs for your blood type: Dong Quai is neutral for people with blood type O, A, B and AB.

Contains: vitamins A, B12 and E, and is very high in iron.

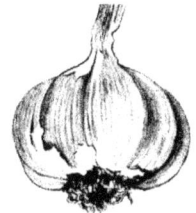

*Garlic

GARLIC can be great for treating the heart. It improves circulation, purifies the blood, and treats infections. It treats digestive disorders, allergies, and asthma. It purifies the blood. **Garlic may elevate blood pressure for some people when taken excessively.** It may be taken in capsules. If it is taken as a tea, use ¼ teaspoon of Garlic herb powder to one cup of boiling water. Garlic may be taken as often as you feel the need. For chronic heart problems it may be taken once or twice a day, for five to seven days, or until the desired results are reached. For some, two or three times a week will be beneficial.

Herbs for your blood type: Garlic is highly beneficial for people with blood type A and AB. It is neutral for people with blood type O and B.

Contains: sodium, sulphur, calcium, copper vitamin B1, iron, and is high in potassium, zinc, selenium, and vitamins A and C.

HEART

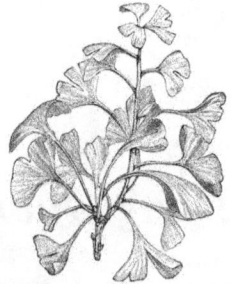

*Ginkgo

GINKGO is excellent for treating the heart. It increases oxygen flow to the heart, treats circulation, edema, blood clots, and helps to prevent strokes. Ginkgo may be taken in capsules. If it is taken as a tea, use ¼ teaspoon of Ginkgo herb powder to one cup of boiling water. Ginkgo may be taken as often as you feel the need. For chronic heart problems it may be taken two or three times a day, for three to seven days, or until desired results are reached. For some, once or twice a week can be beneficial.

Contains bioflavonoids.

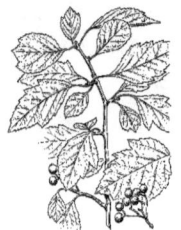

*Hawthorn

HAWTHORN is a great tonic for the heart. It treats cardiac problems, regulates the heart, keeping it from beating to fast or too slow. Hawthorn dilates blood vessels and improves the circulatory system. Hawthorn may be taken in capsules. When it is taken as a tea, use 1/8th teaspoon or less of Hawthorn herb powder to one cup of boiling water. Hawthorn may be taken as often as you feel the need. For chronic heart problems it may be taken once or twice a day for three to five days or until desired results are reached. For some, once or twice a week can be helpful.

Herbs for your blood type: Hawthorn is highly beneficial for people with blood type A and AB. It is neutral for people with blood type O, and B.

Contains: iron, zinc, sodium, sulphur, nickel, tin, aluminum, phosphorus, and a high amount of vitamins C and B complex.

HEART

Kelp

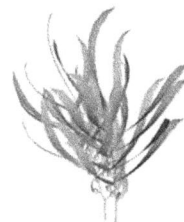

KELP will help to treat diseases of the heart. It cleanses the arteries, removes lead poisoning, and radiation poisoning from the body. Kelp will suppress the appetite and treat obesity. Kelp will help with balancing overactive or under active thyroid glands. Kelp stimulates healthy hair growth. It may be taken in capsules. If it is taken as a tea, use ¼ teaspoon of Kelp herb powder to one cup of boiling water. Kelp may be taken as often as you feel the need. For heart disease it may be taken once or twice a day, for three to five days, or until desired results are reached. For some, once or twice a week will be beneficial.

Contains: calcium, chlorine, sulphur, silicon, zinc, manganese, aluminum, potassium, copper, nickel, iron, silver, phosphorus, vanadium, B complex, vitamins A, C, E, and K, and a very high content of iodine and minerals.

Milk Thistle

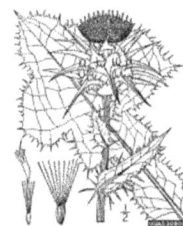

MILK THISTLE can be beneficial for treating the heart. It treats heartburns, hepatitis, nervous conditions, cirrhosis, and helps to soothe the system. Milk Thistle may be taken in capsules. If it is taken as a tea, use ½ teaspoon of Milk Thistle herb powder to one cup of boiling hot water. Milk Thistle may be taken as often as you feel the need. For treating the heart it may be taken once or twice a day, for three to seven days, or until desired results are reached. For some, once or twice a week will be beneficial.

Milk Thistle is high in bioflavonoids.

HEART

*Passion Flower

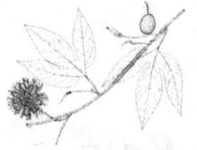

PASSION FLOWER is excellent to use for irregular heartbeat; it treats a weak heart, it offers regularity and strength to the heart. It is a mild sedative for the nerves and will cause sleepiness. It may be taken in capsules, if it is taken as a tea, use ¼ teaspoon of Passion Flower herb powder to one cup of boiling water. Passion Flower may be taken as often as you feel the need. For chronic irregular heartbeat it may be taken once or twice a day, for three to seven days, or until desired results are reached. For some, once or twice a week will be beneficial.

Contains: magnesium and calcium.

*Peppermint

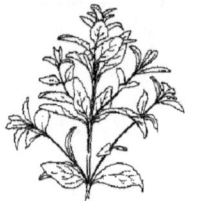

PEPPERMINT is soothing to the heart. It will help to strengthen the heart; treat heart palpitations, heartburn, gas, and indigestion. Peppermint may be taken in capsules. If it is taken as a tea, use ¼ teaspoon of Peppermint herb powder to one cup of boiling water. Peppermint may be taken as often as you feel the need. For chronic heart problems it may be taken once or twice a day, for three to seven days, or until desired results are reached. For some, once or twice a week can be beneficial.

Herbs for your blood type: Peppermint is highly beneficial for people with blood type O and B. It is neutral for people with blood type A and AB.

Contains: iron, niacin, iodine, magnesium, sulphur, potassium, and vitamins A and C.

HEART

*Red Raspberry

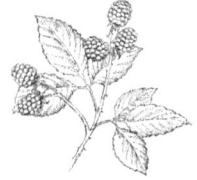

RED RASPBERRY can be excellent for the heart. It helps the heart to become healthy, treats digestive disorders, nausea, and vomiting. Red Raspberry enhances milk in the breast for expectant mothers. Children may use this herb for colds. For children use a smaller amount. It may be taken in capsules, if it is taken as a tea, use ¼ teaspoon of Red Raspberry herb powder to one cup of boiling water. Red Raspberry may be taken as often as you feel the need. For chronic heart problems it may be taken once or twice a day for three to five days, or day until desired results are reached. For some, once or twice a week will be beneficial.

Contains: calcium, manganese, vitamins A, B, C, D, and E, and a very high content of iron.

*Rosemary

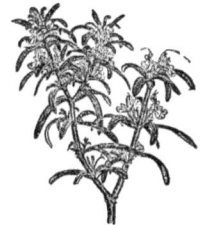

ROSEMARY is an excellent tonic for the heart. It helps with convulsions, muscle spasms, and most stomach disorders. Rosemary treats stress, tension and depression. **Rosemary may elevate blood pressure for some people when taken excessively.** Rosemary may be kept in the kitchen and used as a spice. It may be taken in capsules. If it is taken as a tea, use 1/8th teaspoon, of Rosemary herb powder, to one cup of boiling water. Rosemary may be taken as often as you feel the need. For chronic heart problems it may be taken once or twice a day, for three to five days, or until desired results are reached. For some, once or twice a week will be beneficial.

Contains: iron, sodium, potassium, zinc, phosphorus, magnesium, vitamins A and C, and is high in calcium

---

HEART

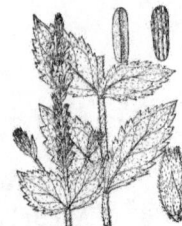

Vervain

VERVAIN will help to strengthen a weak heart. It treats stress, overexertion, asthma, and sleeplessness. Vervain may be taken in capsules. If it is taken as a tea, use ¼ teaspoon of Vervain herb powder to one cup of boiling water. Vervain may be taken as often as you feel the need. For the heart it may be taken once or twice a day, for three to five days, or until desired results are reached. For some, once or twice a week will be beneficial.

Contains: calcium, manganese, vitamins C and E.

HEPATITIS

Astragalus

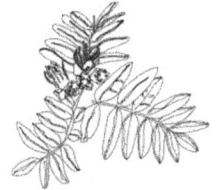

ASTRAGALUS can be helpful for treating hepatitis. It increases strength and vitality, and will enhance the immune system. It treats chronic fatigue, and it heals damaged tissues. Astragalus treats a prolapsed uterus, and eliminates toxins from the system. Astragalus increases white T-cells, and increases urination. It may be taken in capsules. If it is taken as a tea, use ¼ teaspoons of Astragalus herb powder to one cup of boiling water. Astragalus may be taken as often as you feel the need. For hepatitis it may be taken two or three times a day for two to seven days, or until the desired results are reached. For some two or three times a week can be beneficial for prevention.

Contains: choline, betaine, and gluconic acid.

HEPATITIS

HERBS:

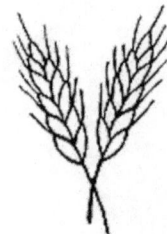

Barley Juice Powder

BARLEY JUICE POWDER can be helpful for treating hepatitis. It is a booster for the immune system, it treats cancer, it neutralizes metals, mercury, and lead in the body. Barley Juice Powder may be taken in capsules. If it is taken as a tea, use ¼ teaspoon of Barley Juice herb powder to one cup of boiling water. Barley Juice Powder may be taken as often as you feel the need. For hepatitis it may be taken once or twice a day, for two to seven days, or until desired results are reached. For some, three or four times a week will be beneficial for prevention.

Contains: vitamins B1, B12, C, potassium, chlorophyll, iron, magnesium, and it is high in calcium.

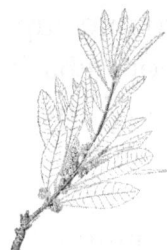

*Bayberry

BAYBERRY is great for treating hepatitis; it has been found to treat a variety of diseases, and is strengthening to the body. Bayberry will help to remove mucus from the lungs. It is a tonic and offers vitality to the body. Bayberry may be taken in capsules. If it is taken as a tea, use ¼ teaspoon of Bayberry herb powder to one cup of boiling water. Bayberry may be taken as often as you feel the need. For chronic hepatitis it may be taken two or three times a day for two to seven days, or until the desired results are reached. For some two or three times a week can be beneficial for prevention.

Contains: potassium, sodium, niacin, calcium, magnesium, manganese, silicon, zinc, vitamins B1, B2, and C.

HEPATITIS

HERBS:

*Dandelion

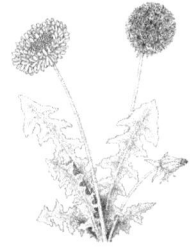

DANDELION is an excellent herb to use for treating hepatitis. It offers endurance, purifies the blood, treats hypoglycemia, and jaundice. Dandelion will stimulate the appetite. **Dandelion may elevate blood pressure for some people when taken excessively.** It may be taken in capsules. If it is taken as a tea, use ¼ teaspoon of Dandelion herb powder to one cup of boiling water. Dandelion may be taken as often as you feel the need. For chronic hepatitis it may be taken two or three times a day for two to seven days, or until desired results are reached. For some, once or twice a week can be beneficial.

Herbs for your blood type: Dandelion is highly beneficial for people with blood type O. It is neutral for people with blood type A, B, and AB.

Contains: calcium, vitamin A, B, C, E, sodium, potassium, iron, nickel, tin copper, magnesium, manganese, sulphur, and zinc.

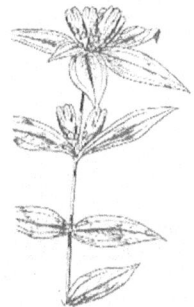

Gentian

GENTIAN can be helpful for treating hepatitis. It is strengthening to the body and it treats exhaustion. Gentian is a tonic and will stimulate the appetite. Buckthorn or Kelp should be taken in combination with this herb. It may be taken in capsules. If it is taken as a tea, use ¼ teaspoon of Gentian herb powder to one cup of boiling water. Gentian may be taken as often as you feel the need. For hepatitis it may be taken once or twice a day, for two to seven days, or until desired results are reached. For some, two or three times a week can be beneficial.

Contains: sulphur, tin, lead, manganese, zinc, and niacin. Gentian is high in iron.

HEPATITIS

HERBS:

Golden Seal

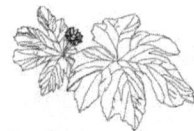

GOLDEN SEAL can offer assistance in treating hepatitis. It is great for treating contagious diseases. It is both an antibiotic and an antiseptic. It treats infections, mouth sores, and typhoid fever. It will reduce sugar in the blood when it is used in combination with the Licorice herb. Use Myrrh with this herb if you suffer from low blood sugar. Do not take this herb if you are pregnant. **Golden Seal may elevate blood pressure for some people.** It may be taken in capsules. If it is taken as a tea, use ¼ teaspoon of Golden Seal herb powder to one cup of boiling water. Golden Seal may be taken as often as you feel the need. For hepatitis it may be taken once or twice a day, for two to seven days, or until desired results are reached. For some, two or three times a week can be beneficial.

Herbs for your blood type: Golden Seal is neutral for people with type A, B and AB. People with blood type O should avoid this herb.

Contains: calcium, potassium, iron, zinc, sodium, and vitamins A, C, B complex, and E.

Horehound:

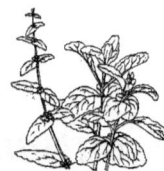

HOREHOUND can help with treating a chronic case of hepatitis. It treats asthma, colds, herpes, hoarseness, phlegm, and tuberculosis. It is highly recommended for relief from lung discomfort. Large amounts of Horehound taken at once will act as a laxative. It may be taken in capsules. If it is taken as a tea, use ¼ teaspoon of Horehound herb powder to one cup of boiling water. Horehound may be taken as often as you feel the need. For chronic hepatitis it may be taken once or twice a day, for two to seven days, or until desired results are reached. For some, once or twice a week can be beneficial.

Herbs for your blood type: Horehound is neutral for people with blood type O, A, B and AB.

Contains: iron, potassium, sulphur, and vitamins A, E, C, and B complex.

HEPATITIS

HERBS:

Lobelia

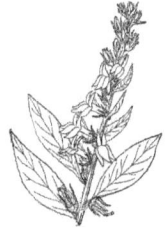

LOBELIA can be excellent for treating hepatitis. It treats contagious diseases, fevers, pain, and pneumonia. Lobelia relaxes the entire system and increases urine flow. It may be taken in capsules. If it is taken as a tea, use ¼ teaspoon of Lobelia herb powder to one cup of boiling water. Lobelia may be taken as often as you feel the need. For hepatitis it may be taken two or three times a day for two to seven days, or until desired results are reached. For some, two or three times a week can be effective.

Contains: iron, copper, sodium, sulphur, cobalt, lead, and selenium.

LOTS OF WATER SHOULD BE TAKEN WITH LOBELIA.

*Milk Thistle

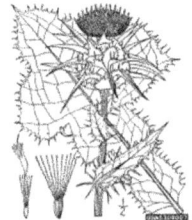

MILK THISTLE is great for treating hepatitis. It treats alcoholism, cirrhosis, and liver problems. Milk Thistle will stimulate the appetite. Milk Thistle may be taken in capsules. If it is taken as a tea, use ½ teaspoon of Milk Thistle herb powder to one cup of boiling hot water. Milk Thistle may be taken as often as you feel the need. For chronic hepatitis it may be taken two or three times a day for two to ten days, or until desired results are reached. For some, two or three times a week can be beneficial.

Milk Thistle is high in bioflavonoids.

HEPATITIS

HERBS:

Oregon Grape

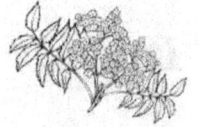

OREGON GRAPE can be helpful for treating hepatitis. It purifies the blood, treats herpes, jaundice, and staph infections. Oregon Grape will stimulate the appetite. Oregon Grape will stimulate the thyroid functions. It cleans the liver. It will increase the immune system while it helps to remedy constipation. Oregon Grape may be taken in capsules. If it is taken as a tea, use ¼ teaspoon of Oregon Grape herb powder to one cup of boiling water. Oregon grape may be taken as often as you feel the need. For hepatitis it may be taken once or twice a day, for two to ten days, or until desired results are reached. For some, two or three times a week can be beneficial.

Contains: sodium, zinc, manganese, copper, and silicon.

Schizandra

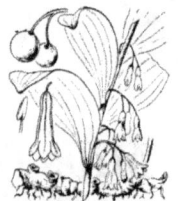

SCHIZANDRA will assist with treating hepatitis. It increases energy, fights fatigue, treats impotency, and offers mental alertness. It helps to improve the functioning of several abdominal organs. It is a tonic for the immune system. **Schizandra may elevate blood pressure for some people when it is taken in a large amount.** It may be taken in capsules. If it is taken as a tea, use ½ teaspoon of Schizandra herb powder to one cup of boiling water. Schizandra may be taken as often as you feel the need. For hepatitis it may be taken once or twice a day, for three to seven days, or until desired results are reached. For some, once or twice a week can be helpful.

Contains: magnesium, calcium, iron, vitamin C, potassium, and sodium.

HEPATITIS

HERBS:

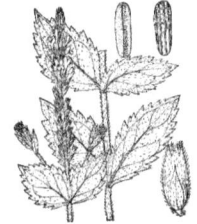

Vervain

VERVAIN can be effective for treating hepatitis. It treats cirrhosis, fevers, jaundice, and tuberculosis. It can be soothing to the system. Vervain should be taken at bedtime,it will cause sleepiness. Vervain may be taken in capsules. If it is taken as a tea, use ¼ teaspoon of Vervain herb powder to one cup of boiling water. Vervain may be taken as often as you feel the need. For hepatitis it may be taken once or twice a day, for two to ten days, or until desired results are reached. For some two or three times a week can be beneficial.

Contains: calcium, manganese, and vitamins C and E.

IMMUNE SYSTEM

HERBS:

Astragalus

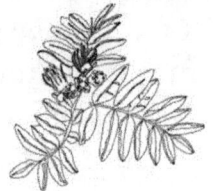

ASTRAGALUS will enhance the immune system. It treats degenerative conditions, and hypertension. Astragalus is excellent to take when you suffer chronic fatigue. It has shown positive effects on cancer patients that are undergoing radiation and chemotherapy treatments. It strengthens the T-cells and helps with chronic lesions. It treats prolapsed organs and uterine cancer. Astragalus will increase urination, it is a diuretic. Astragalus may be taken in capsules. If it is taken as a tea, use ¼ teaspoons of Astragalus herb powder to one cup of boiling water. Astragalus may be taken as often as you feel the need. For treating the immune system it may be taken once or twice a day, for two to seven days, or until desired results are reached. For some, two or three times a week can be beneficial.

Contains: choline, betaine, and gluconic acid.

IMMUNE SYSTEM

HERBS:

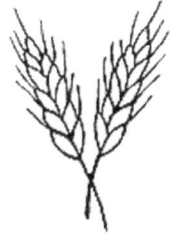

Barley Juice Powder

BARLEY JUICE POWDER will boost the immune system; it treats AIDS, anemia, and cancer. It is great for treating arthritis, metal poisoning, obesity, and other toxic conditions. It can be strengthening to the entire body. Barley Juice Powder may be taken in capsules. If it is taken as a tea, use ¼ teaspoon of Barley Juice Powder to one cup of boiling water.

Barley Juice Powder may be taken as often as you feel the need. For increasing the immune system it may be taken once or twice a day, for two to seven days, or until desired results are reached. For some, two or three times a week will be beneficial.

Contains: vitamins B1, B12, C, potassium, chlorophyll, iron, magnesium, and is high in calcium.

*Bee Propolis

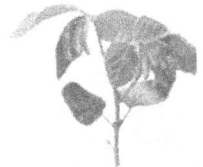

BEE PROPOLIS is excellent for boosting the immune system. It is a stimulant for the immune system; treats pneumonia, respiratory ailments, and shingles. It purifies the blood and stimulates the thymus and thyroid glands. Bee Propolis may be taken in capsules. If it is taken as a tea, use ¼ teaspoon Bee Propolis herb powder to one cup of boiling water. Bee Propolis may be taken as often as you feel the need. For treating the immune system it may be taken once or twice a day, for two to five days, or until desired results are reached. For some, once or twice a week can be beneficial for two to three weeks, or until desired results are reached.

Contains: iron, zinc, copper, magnesium, silicon, and manganese.

IMMUNE SYSTEM

HERBS:

Bilberry

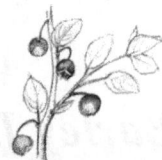

BILBERRY will assist with treating the immune system. It treats infections. It is best known for treating night blindness because it strengthens the capillaries and small veins surrounding the eyes. It treats urinary problems, and can be helpful to strengthen veins during pregnancy. Bilberry may be taken in capsules. If it is taken as a tea use 1/8th teaspoon or less of Bilberry herb powder to one cup of boiling water. Bilberry is best used in combination with other herbs. Bilberry may be taken as often as you feel the need. For treating the immune system it may be taken once or twice a week until desired results are reached.

Contains: manganese, iron, zinc, potassium, calcium, sodium, and selenium.

*Echinacea

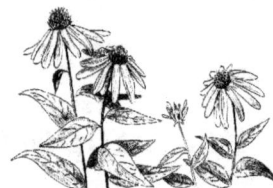

ECHINACEA is stimulating to the immune system. It treats immune deficiency, it cleans the lymphatic system and purifies the blood. It treats the prostate glands and treats syphilis. Echinacea is an antibiotic and it increases white blood cells. It may be taken in capsules. If it is taken as tea, use ¼ teaspoon of Echinacea herb powder to one cup of boiling water. Echinacea may be taken as often as you feel the need. For the immune system it may be taken once or twice a day, for two to five days, or until desired results are reached. For some, once or twice a week can be beneficial.

Herbs for your blood type: Echinacea is highly beneficial for people with blood type A and AB. It is neutral for people with blood type B. People with blood type O should avoid this herb. Echinacea will cause excessive blood thinning for people with blood type O.

Contains: vitamins A, C, E, iron, iodine, copper, sulphur, and potassium.

IMMUNE SYSTEM

*Pau D'Arco

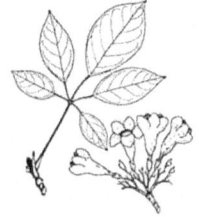

PAU D' ARCO is excellent for treating the immune system. It increases the immune system, treats immune deficiency, and has the ability to reduce and dissolve tumors. It has great cancer fighting abilities as well. Pau D'Arco may be taken in capsules. If it is taken as a tea, use ¼ teaspoon of Pau D'Arco herb powder to one cup of boiling water. Pau D'Arco may be taken as often as you feel the need. For the immune system it may be taken once or twice a week until desired results are reached.

Contains: potassium, sodium, magnesium, manganese, selenium, zinc, vitamins A, B complex, and C, and is very high in iron.

*Suma

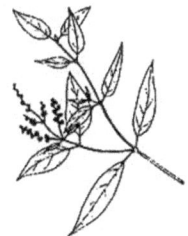

SUMA strengthens the immune system. It increases energy, reduces tumors, treats leukemia, and Hodgkin's disease. Suma increases vitality. It may be taken in capsules. If it is taken as a tea, use ¼ teaspoon of Suma herb powder to one cup of boiling water. Suma may be taken as often as you feel the need. For treating the immune system it may be taken once or twice a day, for two to five days, or until desired results are reached. For some, two or three times a week can be beneficial for desired results.

Contains: iron, magnesium, vitamin B complex, minerals, and amino acids.

KIDNEY

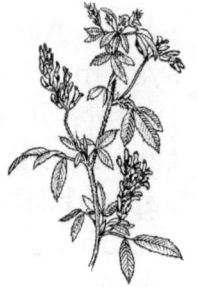

Alfalfa

ALFALFA will work to clean the kidneys. It treats liver conditions, peptic ulcers, and tooth decay. It stimulates the appetite, purifies the blood, and neutralizes acidity. Alfalfa helps to prevent colon cancer when taken over an extended period of time. Alfalfa it may be taken in capsules. If it is taken as a tea, use ¼ teaspoon of Alfalfa herb powder to one cup of boiling water. Alfalfa may be taken as often as you feel the need. For cleaning the kidneys it may be taken two or three times a day, for two to seven days, or until desired results are reached. For some, two or three times a week can be beneficial.

Herbs for your blood type: Alfalfa is highly beneficial for people with blood type A. And it is neutral for people with blood type B and AB. People with blood type O should avoid this herb it will cause excessive blood thinning for them.

Contains: vitamins A, B complex, D, E, K, iron, potassium, magnesium, protein, sodium, sulfur, and phosphorus. Alfalfa is very high in calcium, chlorophyll, and vitamin B12.

KIDNEY

Amaranth

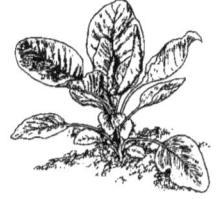

AMARANTH can assist with treating the kidneys. It treats diarrhea, herpes, and excessive menstruation. It treats several viruses and bleeding gums. Amaranth may be taken in capsules. If it is taken as a tea, use ½ teaspoon of Amaranth herb powder to one cup of boiling water. Amaranth may be taken as often as you feel the need. For treating the kidneys it may be taken once or twice a day, for three to seven days, or until desired results are reached. For some, three or four times a week can be helpful.

Contains: vitamin C, magnesium, potassium, niacin, and is very high in protein, iron, calcium, and has a high concentration of amino acid L-Lysine.

Astragalus

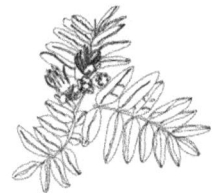

ASTRAGALUS can be helpful with treating the kidneys. It gives support to the liver, and strengthens the digestive system. Astragalus strengthens T-cells and helps to lower blood pressure. Urination will increase while using this herb. It treats prolapsed organs and uterine cancer. It may be taken in capsules. If it is taken as a tea, use ¼ teaspoon of Astragalus herb powder to one cup of boiling water. Astragalus may be taken as often as you feel the need. For treating the kidneys it may be taken two or three times a day for three to seven days, or until the desired results are reached. For some, once or twice a week can be helpful.

Contains: choline, betaine, and gluconic acid.

KIDNEY

HERBS:

Barberry

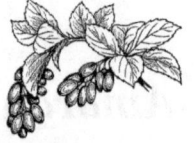

BARBERRY can lend assistance in treating the kidneys. It treats serious liver conditions and jaundice. Barberry works best when used in combination with other herbs. **Do not take Barberry excessively; it may cause depression.** It dilates blood vessels, which makes it a good treatment for high blood pressure. Barberry may be taken in capsules. If it is taken as a tea, use 1/8th teaspoon of Barberry herb powder to one cup of boiling water. Barberry may be taken as often as you feel the need. For treating kidney problems it may be taken once or twice a day, for two to seven days, or until desired results are reached. For some, once or twice a week can be helpful.

Contains: iron, manganese, phosphorus, and vitamin C.

Barley Juice Powder

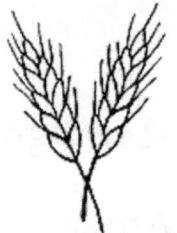

BARLEY JUICE POWDER will help to repair the kidneys. It will boost the immune system, purify the blood and will assist with treating cancer. Barley Juice Powder will help to remove lead and mercury from the body. It may be taken in capsules. If it is taken as a tea, use ¼ teaspoon of Barley Juice herb Powder to one cup of boiling water. Barley Juice Powder may be taken as often as you feel the need. For kidney problems it may be taken once a day for two to seven days, or until desired results are reached. For some, once or twice a week can be helpful until desired results are reached.

Contains: vitamins B1, B12, C, potassium, chlorophyll, iron, magnesium, and is high in calcium.

KIDNEY

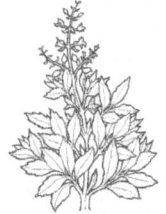

Basil

BASIL can assist with treating the kidneys. It treats bladder and liver problems, and helps to eliminate parasites from the body. Basil is best-used fresh in salads and other food preparations. Basil can be taken in capsules. If it is taken as a tea, use ¼ teaspoon of Basil herb powder to one cup of boiling water. Basil may be taken as often as you feel the need. For treating the kidneys it may be taken once or twice a day, for two to seven days, or until desired results are reached. For some, once or twice a week can be helpful.

   Herbs for your blood type: Basil is neutral for people with blood type O, A, B, and AB.

Contains: iron, calcium, magnesium, phosphorus, and vitamins A, D, and B2.

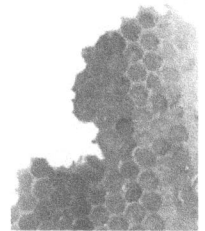

Bee's Royal Jelly

BEE'S ROYAL JELLY will assist with treating diseased kidneys. It will boost the immune system and offers increased stamina. Bee's Royal Jelly will treat insomnia and prostate problems. It is high in all of the B vitamins as well as minerals. Bee's Royal Jelly is best taken at bedtime. It may be taken in capsules, if it is taken as a tea, use ¼ teaspoon of Bee's Royal Jelly herb powder to one cup of boiling water. Bee's Royal Jelly may be taken as often as you feel the need. For diseased kidneys it may be taken once or twice a day, for two to ten days, or until desired results are reached. For some, once or twice a week can be helpful.

Bee's Royal Jelly is high in all of the B vitamins and minerals.

HERBS TO HELP YOU HEAL

KIDNEY

Birch

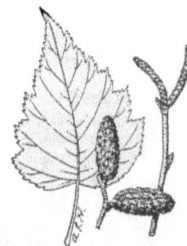

BIRCH is a good choice to use for treating the kidneys. It removes kidney stones and is excellent for treating the bladder and urinary tract disorders. Birch cleans the blood and treats cancer. Birch is a diuretic and a sedative. Birch may be taken at bedtime for insomnia. It may be taken in capsules. If it is taken as a tea, use ¼ teaspoon of Birch herb powder to one cup of boiling water. Birch may be taken as often as you feel the need. For treating the kidneys it may be taken once or twice a day, for two to seven days, or until desired results are reached. For some, once or twice a week will give results over an extended period of time.

Contains: copper, sodium, calcium, iron, magnesium, potassium, silicon, vitamin A, B1, B2, C, and E.

Black Cohosh

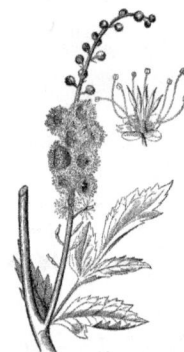

BLACK COHOSH can be helpful for treating the kidneys. It treats the liver and all types of inflammation in the joints. It cleans the blood and treats chronic bronchitis. **Black Cohosh is a sedative; it should be used in small amounts or it can cause a headache.** Black Cohosh lowers the heart rate slightly but increases the pulse rate. Black Cohosh may be taken in capsules. If it is taken as a tea, use 1/8th teaspoon or less of Black Cohosh herb powder, to one cup of boiling water. Black Cohosh may be taken as often as you feel the need. For treating the kidneys it may be taken once a day, for to five days, or until desired results are reached. For some, once or twice a week can be helpful.

Contains: calcium, potassium, iron, magnesium, manganese, niacin, phosphorus, selenium, silicon, sodium, sulphur, vitamins A, B1, B2, C, K, and F, and zinc.

KIDNEY

HERBS:

Blessed Thistle

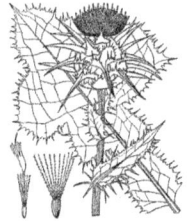

BLESSED THISTLE can be useful for treating the kidneys. It treats the liver, gallbladder, and poor circulation. It treats angina, and cancer, purifies the blood, and stimulates the brain. Blessed Thistle may be taken in capsules. If it is taken as a tea, use ¼ teaspoon of Blessed Thistle herb to one cup of boiling water. Blessed Thistle may be taken as often as you feel the need. For treating the kidneys it may be taken once or twice a day, for two to ten days, or until desired results are reached. For some, once or twice a week can give results in a short period.

Contains: B complex, calcium, iron, manganese, and potassium.

*Buchu

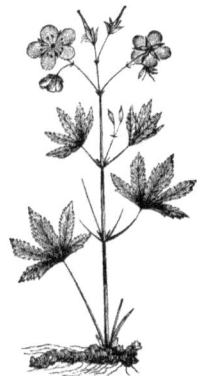

BUCHU is excellent for treating the kidneys. It treats chronic kidney inflammation and kidney stones. It relieves back pain and treats urinary infections. It will assist with lowering blood pressure. Urination increases while using Buchu. It may be taken in capsules. If it is taken as a tea, use ¼ teaspoon of Buchu herb powder to one cup of boiling water. Buchu may be taken as often as you feel the need. For chronic kidney problems it may be taken two or three times a day, for two to five days, or until desired results are reached. For some, once or twice a week will be beneficial for two to three weeks.

Contains bioflavonoids.

KIDNEY

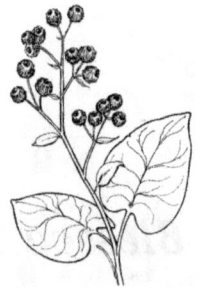

*Burdock

BURDOCK is excellent for treating chronic issues with the kidneys. It can be useful for promoting kidney function, and it removes inflammation from the liver. Burdock is excellent for treating cancer, and it purifies the blood. It treats infections in the bladder, constipation, and fluid retention. It may be taken in capsules. If it is taken as a tea, use ¼ teaspoon of Burdock herb powder to one cup of boiling water. Burdock may be taken as often as you feel the need. For chronic kidney problems it may be taken once or twice a day, for two to seven days, or until desired results are reached. For some once or twice a week will be beneficial. Do not use an excessive amount of Burdock at once it may cause vomiting.

Herbs for your blood type: Burdock is highly beneficial for people with blood type A and AB. It is neutral for people with blood type B. People with blood type O should avoid this herb it will cause excessive blood thinning and excessive bleeding for people with blood type O.

Contains: vitamins A. E. P. and B complex, sulphur, silicon, copper, iodine, zinc, and is rich in vitamin C and iron.

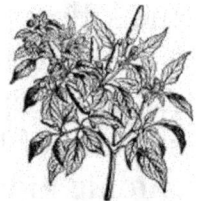

Capsicum/ Cayenne

CAPSICUM/ CAYENNE can assist with treating the kidneys. It treats infections, inflammation of the kidneys, and stimulates circulation. Capsicum/ Cayenne has a hot peppery taste and it may be taken in capsules. If it is taken as a tea, use 1/8th teaspoon of capsicum/cayenne herb powder to one cup of boiling water. Capsicum/ Cayenne may be taken as often as you feel the need. For treating the kidneys it may be taken once or twice a day, for two to seven days, or until the desired results are reached. For some two or three times a week can be helpful.

KIDNEY

HERBS:

Herbs for your blood type: Capsicum/Cayenne is highly beneficial for people with blood type O. It is neutral for people with blood B and AB. People with blood type A should avoid this herb.

Contains: vitamins A, C, magnesium, and sulphur. Capsicum/Cayenne is very high in iron, potassium, and calcium.

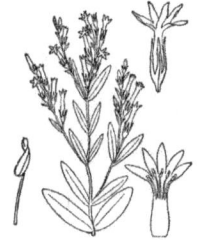

*Centaury

CENTAURY is excellent for strengthen the kidneys. It is also very effective for treating the bladder, liver problems, and increasing the appetite. **Pregnant women should avoid the use Centaury; it will not be safe for baby.** Centaury may be taken in capsules. If it is taken as a tea, use ¼ teaspoon of Centaury herb powder to one cup of boiling water. Centaury may be taken as often as you feel the need. For treating chronic kidney problems it may be taken once or twice a day, for three or four days, or until desired results are reached. For some, once or twice a week can be beneficial.

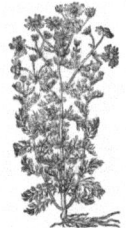

Chamomile

CHAMOMILE helps to stimulate the kidneys; it also treats the bladder, the spleen, and it stimulates and cleans the liver. It treats poor circulation and fevers. Chamomile is best known for treating nervous disorders. It will increases the appetite. Chamomile is best taken at bedtime. Chamomile can be taken in capsules, if it is taken as a tea, use ¼ teaspoon of Chamomile herb powder to one cup of boiling water. Chamomile may be taken as often as you feel the need. For treating the kidneys it may be taken once or twice a day, for two to seven days, or until desired results are reached. For some, two or three times a week can be beneficial until desired results are reached.

Herbs for your blood type: Chamomile is highly beneficial for people with blood type A and AB. It is neutral for people with blood type O, and B.

Contains: potassium, calcium, iron, manganese, vitamin A, and zinc.

KIDNEY

Chicory

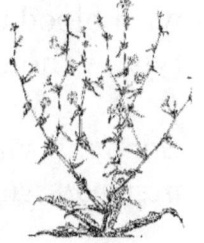

CHICORY can be useful for treating the kidneys. It will purify and clean the blood. It treats jaundice, liver problems, and it helps to relieve stiff joints. Chicory will help to remove calcium deposits from the body. It may be taken in capsules, if it is taken as a tea, use ¼ teaspoon of Chicory herb powder to one cup of boiling water. Chicory may be taken as often as you feel the need. For treating the kidneys it may be taken once or twice a day, for two to five days, or until desired results are reached. For some, once or twice a week can be beneficial.

Contains: a high amount of vitamins A, B, C, K, and P.

Comfrey

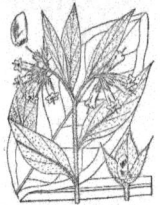

COMFREY can be helpful for treating stones in the kidneys. It treats bloody urine, infections, and breathing problems such as asthma and emphysema. Comfrey stimulates new cell growth and provides healing for the body. It promotes healthy skin. Comfrey may be taken in capsules. If it is taken as a tea, use ¼ teaspoon of Comfrey herb powder to one cup of boiling water. Comfrey may be taken as often as you feel the need. For treating the kidneys it may be taken two or three times a day, for two to seven days, or until desired results are reached. For some, two or three times a week can be helpful for prevention.

Contains: vitamins A, C, iron, sulphur, copper, zinc, and magnesium. Comfrey is very high in calcium, potassium, and protein.

KIDNEY

*Couch Grass

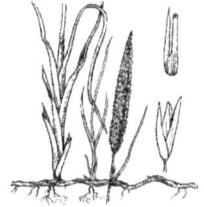

COUCH GRASS can be very beneficial for treating the kidneys. It treats bladder infections, jaundice, and urinary infections. It treats female disorders, enlarged prostate glands, and syphilis. It may be taken in capsules. If it is taken as a tea, use ¼ teaspoon of Couch Grass herb powder to one cup of boiling water. Couch Grass may be taken as often as you feel the need. For chronic kidney problems it may be taken two or three times a day, for two to seven days, or until desired results are reached. For some, two or three times a week will be beneficial.

Contains: vitamin A, C, B complex, sodium, potassium, calcium, and magnesium. Couch Grass has a high amount of silicon,

Damiana

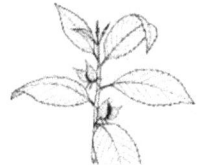

DAMIANA will assist with treating the kidneys. It treats inflammation in the kidneys, and the bladder, it treats pulmonary disorders, emphysema, and it helps to overcome exhaustion. Damiana is an aphrodisiac and will enhance sexual desires in both men and women. It may be taken in capsules. If it is taken as a tea, use ¼ teaspoon of Damiana herb powder to one cup of boiling water. Damiana may be taken as often as you feel the need. For treating the kidneys it may be taken once or twice a day, for two to five days, or until desired results are reached. For some, once or twice a week can be helpful.

Contains: vitamins A and C, zinc, B complex, calcium, potassium, protein, selenium, and sodium.

KIDNEY

HERBS:

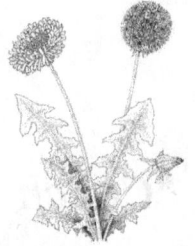

*Dandelion

DANDELION can be excellent for treating the kidneys; it treats infection in the kidneys, jaundice, and liver disorders. Dandelion offers endurance. **Dandelion may elevate blood pressure for some people when taken excessively.** It may be taken in capsules. If it is taken as a tea, use ¼ teaspoon of Dandelion herb powder to one cup of boiling water. Dandelion may be taken as often as you feel the need. For treating the kidneys it may be taken once or twice a day, for two to seven days, or until desired results are reached. For some, two or three times a week can be helpful.

Herbs for your blood type: Dandelion is highly beneficial for people with blood type O. It is neutral for people with blood type A, B, and AB.

Contains: calcium, vitamins A, B, C, and E, sodium, potassium, iron, nickel, tin, copper, magnesium, manganese, sulphur, and zinc.

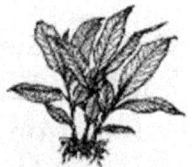

*Devil's Claw

DEVIL'S CLAW is an excellent herb to strengthen the kidneys. It strengthens the bladder, purifies the blood, and treats liver diseases. It reduces inflammation in the joints and strengthens the whole system while it works. Devil's Claw may be taken in capsules. If it is taken as a tea, use ¼ teaspoon of Devil's Claw herb powder to one cup of boiling water. Devil's Claw may be taken as often as you feel the need. For chronic kidney problems it may be taken once or twice a day, for two to seven days, or until desired results are reached. For some, once or twice a week can be beneficial.

Contains: Calcium, iron, magnesium, manganese, phosphorus, potassium, protein, selenium, silicon, sodium, and vitamins A, C, and zinc.

KIDNEY

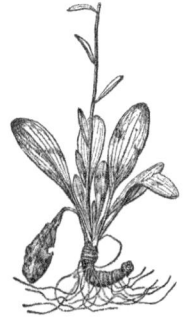

*False Unicorn

FALSE UNICORN can be great for treating the kidneys. It treats uterine problems, prostate problems, and prolapsed uterus. False Unicorn has been known to prevent miscarriages. It has been used with success for treating infertility. It is a tonic that will help with male impotency. It may be taken in capsules. If it is taken as a tea, use ¼ teaspoon of false unicorn herb powder to one cup of boiling water. False Unicorn may be taken as often as you feel the need. For treating the kidneys it may be taken once or twice a day for two to ten days, or a day until desired results are reached. For some, two or three times a week will be beneficial.

Contains: vitamin C, copper, sulphur, and some zinc.

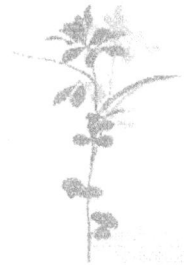

Fenugreek

FENUGREEK can offer assistance for the kidneys. It treats and lubricates inflamed intestines. Fenugreek helps to lower blood sugar. It treats allergies and stomach irritations. **Fenugreek should not be used by women who wish to get pregnant it will impede the progress.** Fenugreek may be taken in capsules. If it is taken as a tea, use ¼ teaspoon of Fenugreek herb powder to one cup of boiling water. Fenugreek may be taken as often as you feel the need. For treating the kidneys it may be taken once or twice a day for two to seven days, or until desired results are reached. For some, two or three times a week can offer assistance.

Herbs for your blood type: Fenugreek is highly beneficial for people with blood type O, and A. People with blood type B, or AB should avoid this herb.

Contains: B1, B2, iron, and choline, and is very high in vitamins A and D.

KIDNEY

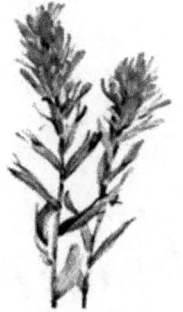

Figwort

FIGWORT helps to maintain and clean the kidneys. It treats liver problems and skin diseases. **Do not use Figwort during pregnancy it promotes menstruation.** Figwort should be taken at bedtime, it will promote sleep. It is a diuretic. Figwort may be taken in capsules. If it is taken as a tea, use ¼ teaspoon of Figwort herb powder to one cup of boiling water. Figwort may be taken as often as you feel the need. For treating the kidneys it may be taken once or twice a day for two to five days, or until desired results are reached. For some, once or twice a week can be helpful.

Content: vitamin information unknown.

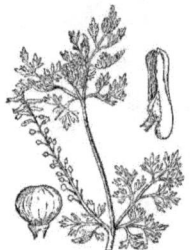

*Fumitory

FUMITORY will remove inflammation from the kidneys. It treats chronic kidney, and liver congestion. Fumitory acts as a laxative and is a diuretic. It will help to lower high blood pressure. Use this herb sparingly or it will cause stomach cramps. Fumitory may be taken in capsules. If it is taken as a tea, use1/8th teaspoon or less of Fumitory herb powder to one cup of boiling water. Fumitory may be taken as often as you feel the need. For treating kidneys it may be taken once a day for two to five days, or until desired results are reached. For some, once a week can be helpful.

Content: vitamin information unknown.

KIDNEY

Garlic

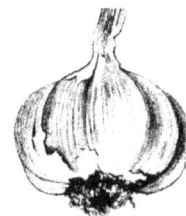

GARLIC can be helpful for treating the kidneys. It promotes kidney functions, detoxifies the liver, and treats the lungs. It has cancer-fighting properties. It treats poor circulation, and chronic bronchitis. **Garlic may elevate blood pressure for some people when taken excessively.** Garlic may be taken in capsules, if it is taken as a tea, use ¼ teaspoon of Garlic herb powder to one cup of boiling water. Garlic may be taken as often as you feel the need. For treating the kidneys it may be taken once or twice a day, for two to five days, or until desired results are reached. For some, once or twice a week can be helpful.

Herbs for your blood type: Garlic is highly beneficial for people with blood type A and AB. It is neutral for people with blood type O and B.

Contains: sodium, sulphur, calcium, copper, vitamin B1, and iron. Garlic is high in potassium, zinc, selenium, and vitamins A and C.

Ginger

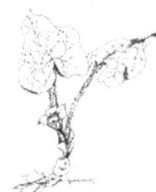

GINGER will help with treating the kidneys. It will increase urine flow. It prevents blood clotting and lowers cholesterol. It improves circulation throughout the body. Do not take aspirins while using Ginger; it will inhibit the performance. It is best found in the produce section of the grocery market. Ginger may be taken in capsules. If it is taken as a tea, grate the ginger and steep it in a container with a covered lid. Ginger may be taken as often as you feel the need. For treating kidneys it may be taken once or twice a day, for two to seven days, or until desired results are reached. For some, two or three times a week will can be helpful.

Herbs for your blood type: Ginger is highly beneficial for people with blood type O, A, B and AB.

Contains: vitamins A, B complex, C, calcium, iron, sodium, potassium, and magnesium.

KIDNEY

HERBS:

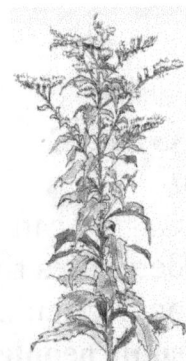

Golden Rod

GOLDEN ROD can assist with treating the kidneys. It clears up dark cloudy urine, and removes kidney stones. It treats urinary problems, such as stones in the bladder. Golden Rod is a diuretic. It may be taken in capsules. If it is taken as tea, use ¼ teaspoon of Golden Rod herb powder to one cup of boiling water. Golden Rod may be taken as often as you feel the need. For treating kidneys it may be taken once or twice a day, for two to seven days, or until desired results are reached. For some, once or twice a week can be beneficial.

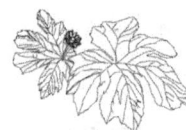

*Golden Seal

GOLDEN SEAL is excellent for treating kidney problems, such as chronic infections and inflammation of the kidneys. Golden Seal will reduce sugar in the blood when used with the Licorice herb Myrrh should be used with this herb if there is low blood sugar. Pregnant women should not use this herb during pregnancy. **Golden Seal may elevate blood pressure for some people when taken excessively.** Golden Seal may be taken in capsules. If it is taken as a tea, use ¼ teaspoon of Golden Seal herb powder to one cup of boiling water. Golden Seal may be taken as often as you feel the need. For treating chronic kidney problems it may be taken two or three times a day, for two to seven days, or until desired results are reached. For some, two or three times a week will be beneficial.

Herbs for your blood type: Golden Seal is neutral for people with blood type A, B and AB. People with blood type O should avoid this herb.

Contains: calcium, potassium, iron, zinc, sodium, and vitamins A, C, B complex, and E.

KIDNEY
---

*Horsetail

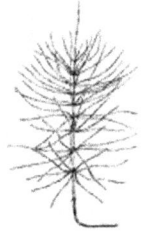

HORSETAIL removes stones from the kidneys, and treats overactive liver problems. Horsetail treats bladder problems and increases urination. It eliminates urinary ulcers and diabetes. Horsetail is excellent for hair and fingernail growth. **People with high blood pressure should not take Horsetail more than once a week.** It may be taken in capsules. If it is taken as a tea, use ¼ teaspoon of Horsetail herb powder to one cup of boiling water. Horsetail may be taken as often as you feel the need. For treating the kidneys it may be taken once or twice a day for two to seven days or until desired results are reached. For some, two or three times a week can be beneficial.

Contains: sodium, iron, iodine, copper and vitamin E, and a high amount of silicon and selenium.

Hyssop

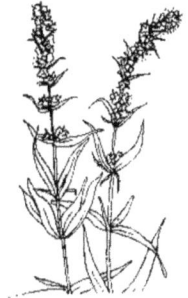

HYSSOP will assist with treating the kidneys. It treats problems with the liver, strengthens the immune system, and will help to lower blood pressure. It will do wonders to soothe the wheezing associated with asthma. Hyssop may be taken in capsules. If it is taken as a tea, use ¼ teaspoon of Hyssop herb powder to one cup of boiling water. Hyssop may be taken as often as you feel the need. For treating the kidneys it may be taken once or twice a day, for two to seven days, or until desired results are reached. For some, once or twice a week can be helpful.

Contains: nutrients of sulfur, flavonoids, marrubin, and tannins.

KIDNEY

*Juniper

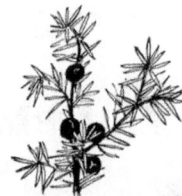

JUNIPER clears up infections of the kidneys; it removes stones from the kidneys. Do not use Juniper internally if you suffer from kidney disease; it may over stimulate the kidneys. It is great for treating bladder problems. It treats burning urination and chronic urinary problems. **Juniper is not recommended for pregnant women.** Juniper produces natural insulin in the body. It may be taken in capsules. If it is taken as a tea, use ¼ teaspoon of Juniper herb powder to one cup of boiling water. Juniper may be taken as often as you feel the need. For treating chronic kidney problems it may be taken once or twice a day, for two to seven days, or until desired results are reached. For some, two or three times a week can be beneficial.

Contains: sulphur, copper, a high amount of vitamin C, and a small amount of aluminum.

Kelp

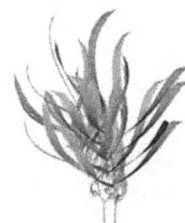

KELP can be useful for treating the kidneys. It increases vitality, treats tumors, and removes lead poisoning from the body. Kelp helps the brain to function normally. It is excellent for nails and hair health. Kelp affects the thyroid by balancing overactive, or under active thyroid glands. Kelp may be taken in capsules. If it is taken as a tea, use ¼ teaspoon of Kelp herb powder to one cup of boiling water. Kelp may be taken as often as you feel the need. For treating the kidneys it may be taken once a day for two to five days, or until desired results are reached. For some, once or twice a week will be beneficial.

Contains: calcium, chlorine, sulphur, silicon, zinc, manganese, aluminum, potassium, copper, nickel, iron, silver, phosphorus, vanadium, B complex, and vitamins A, C, E, and K, it has a very high content of iodine and minerals.

KIDNEY

*Marshmallow

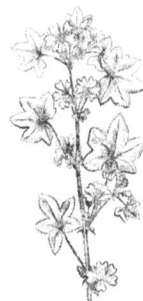

MARSHMALLOW is excellent for treating the kidneys; it works great for removing kidney stones from the body. It treats inflammation from the urinary tract and stops painful urination. **Marshmallow may elevate blood pressure for some people when taken excessively.** Marshmallow may be taken in capsules. If it is taken as a tea, use ¼ teaspoon of Marshmallow herb powder to one cup of boiling water. Marshmallow may be taken as often as you feel the need. For treating the kidneys it may be taken once or twice a day for two to seven days, or until desired results are reached. For some, two or three times a week can be beneficial.

Do not confuse Marshmallow herb with the candy like marshmallow found in the food section of the market.

Contains: sodium, iodine, B complex, pantothenic acid, and is high in calcium, zinc, and iron.

Nettle

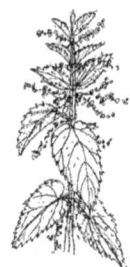

NETTLE will treat an inflamed kidney. It treats urinary infections, increases blood circulation, and will increase the thyroid function. Nettle treats scalp infections, and baldness. Nettle may be taken in capsules. If it is taken as a tea, use ¼ teaspoon of Nettle herb powder to one cup of boiling water. Nettle may be taken as often as you feel the need. For inflamed kidneys it may be taken once a day for two to ten days, or until desired results are reached. For some, once or twice a week can be helpful.

Contains: vitamins A, C, D, E, F, and P, copper, potassium, sodium, calcium, chlorophyll, sulphur, silicon, protein, and zinc, and is high in iron and minerals.

KIDNEY

HERBS:

Oregon Grape

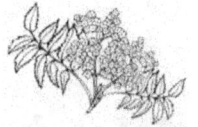

OREGON GRAPE can be helpful for treating the kidneys. It purifies the blood and cleans the lymphatic system. Oregon Grape will stimulate the thyroid functions. It cleans the liver organs and strengthens the immune system. It offers a laxative effect, it has antiseptic qualities, and stimulates the appetite. Oregon Grape may be taken in capsules. If it is taken as a tea, use ¼ teaspoon of Oregon Grape herb powder to one cup of boiling water. Oregon Grape may be taken as often as you feel the need. For treating the kidneys it may be taken once or twice a day, for two to seven days, or until desired results are reached. For some, two or three times a week can be beneficial.

Contains: sodium, zinc, manganese, copper, and silicon.

*Peach Bark

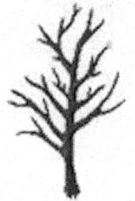

PEACH BARK is excellent for treating the kidneys. It works great at treating bladder and urinary problems. It treats burning in the urine, and stimulates the flow of urine. It helps to relieve gas and colic, and treats the mucus membrane. **Pregnant women should not take Peach Bark, it can induce miscarriage.** Peach Bark may be taken in capsules. If it is taken as a tea, use ¼ teaspoon of Peach Bark herb powder to one cup of boiling water. Peach Bark may be taken as often as you feel the need. For treating chronic kidney problems it may be taken once or twice a day, for two to ten days, or until desired results are reached. For some, once or twice a week can be beneficial.

Content: vitamin information unknown.

KIDNEY

HERBS:

*Plantain

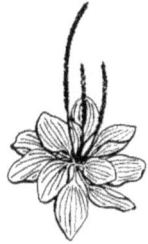

PLANTAIN is a great herb to use for treating the kidneys. It treats incontinence and it is excellent for treating bladder and urinary infections. Plantain suppresses the appetite and lowers cholesterol. It may be used as a poultice on the back for pain. Plantain may be taken in capsules. If it is taken as a tea, use ¼ teaspoon of Plantain herb powder to one cup of boiling water. Plantain may be taken as often as you feel the need. For chronic kidney problems it may be taken once or twice a day, for two to ten days, or until desired results are reached. For some once or twice a week can be beneficial.

Contains: a high amount of vitamins C, K, calcium, sulphur, potassium, and is high in minerals.

Pleurisy Root

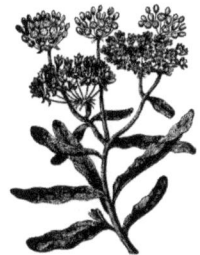

PLEURISY ROOT can be helpful for treating the kidneys. It increases urinary functions and treats water retention, Pleurisy Root will increase perspiration. It will also remove mucus from the respiratory system. It will expel gas and relieve colic. **Do not use Pleurisy Root with a weak pulse and cold skin. Yarrow may be used instead. Pleurisy Root is not recommended for children. It may cause vomiting when taken excessively. Do not use Pleurisy during pregnancy it may induce spontaneous abortion. Do not use while breast-feeding. Large amounts of Pleurisy Root may be very toxic. Do not use Pleurisy if there is a history of heart disease, or certain types of cancer.** Pleurisy Root relaxes the whole body. Vitamin C should be taken when using this herb. It may be taken in capsules, if it is taken as a tea, use 1/8th teaspoon or less of Pleurisy Root herb powder to one cup of boiling water. Use Pleurisy under supervision of a health provider. Pleurisy Root may be taken as often as you feel the need. For treating the kidneys it may be taken once a day for two to three days, or until desired results are reached. For some, once or twice a week can be helpful.

KIDNEY

HERBS:

Content: vitamin information unknown.

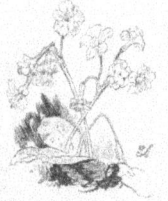

*Queen of the Meadow

QUEEN OF THE MEADOW is excellent for treating the kidneys. It treats gravel, infections, prostate glands, and uterine disease. It will allow an easy urine flow when there is a chronic problem. It may be taken in capsules. If it is taken as a tea, use ¼ teaspoon of Queen of The Meadow herb powder to one cup of boiling water. Queen of The Meadow may be taken as often as you feel the need. For kidney infections it may be taken once or twice a day, for two to five days, or until desired results are reached. For some once or twice a week can be beneficial.

Contains: vitamins A, C, and D.

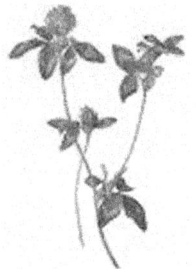

Red Clover

RED CLOVER can be helpful for treating the kidneys. It treats urinary problems, chronic bladder problems, cancer, and liver congestion. It has a laxative effect on the system. It is a tonic and will calm the nerves and increase energy. It may be taken in capsules, if it is taken as a tea, use ¼ teaspoon of Red Clover herb powder to one cup of boiling water. Red Clover may be taken as often as you feel the need. For kidney problems it may be taken once a day for two to five days, or until desired results are reached. For some, once or twice a week can be helpful.

Contains: vitamins A, B complex, calcium, sodium, nickel, manganese, and tin.

KIDNEY

HERBS:

Rose Hips

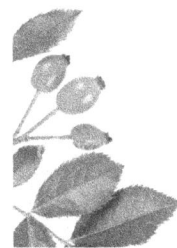

ROSE HIPS can be useful for treating the kidneys. It treats kidney stones and exhaustion. It is an excellent cancer treatment. It can also be helpful for people that is allergic to citrus. Rose Hips is an excellent alternative to vitamin C. Rose Hips may be taken in capsules. If it is taken as a tea, use ¼ teaspoon of Rose Hips herb powder to one cup of boiling water. Rose Hips may be taken as often as you feel the need. For treating the kidneys it may be taken once or twice a day, for two to five days, or until desired results are reached. For some, three or four times a week will be helpful.

Herbs for your blood type: Rose Hips is highly beneficial for people with blood type O, A, B, and AB.

Contains: iron, sodium, sulphur, potassium, niacin, vitamins A, B complex, C, and E, and is very high in vitamin C.

Sage

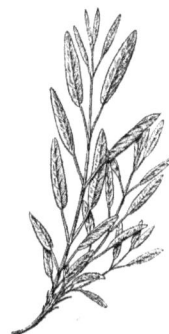

SAGE can be helping for treating the kidneys. It treats the liver, bladder infections, and baldness. Sage will improve memory and treat nausea. Sage may be taken in capsules. If it is taken as a tea, use ¼ teaspoon of Sage herb powder to one cup of boiling water. Sage may be taken as often as you feel the need. For treating the kidneys it may be taken once or twice a day, for two to five days, or until the desired results are reached.

Herbs for your blood type: Sage is highly beneficial for people with blood type B. It is neutral for people with blood type O, A, and AB.

Contains: sodium, sulphur, vitamins A, B complex, and C.

KIDNEY

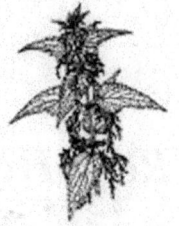

Saw Palmetto

SAW PALMETTO will help to treat diseased kidneys. It treats bladder and urinary infections. Saw Palmetto is a sexual stimulant that treats frigidity and impotency. It will also reduce enlarged prostate glands. Saw Palmetto may be taken in capsules. If it is taken as a tea, use ¼ teaspoon of Saw Palmetto herb powder to one cup of boiling water. Saw Palmetto may be taken as often as you feel the need. For treating the kidneys it may be taken once a day for two to seven days, or until desired results are reached. For some, once or twice a week on and off until you reach the desired results.

Contains vitamin A.

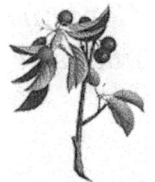

*Uva Ursi

UVA URSI is excellent for treating the kidneys. It treats infections in the kidneys, and kidney stones. It treats liver problems, gallstones, and urinary disorders. **Do not use large quantities of this herb during pregnancy; it could decrease circulation to the fetus.** Uva Ursi increases the flow of urine and acts as a disinfectant. Uva Ursi will turn the urine a dark green do not panic it is normal. Uva Ursi may be taken in capsules. If it is taken as a tea, use ¼ teaspoon of Uva Ursi to one cup of boiling water. Uva Ursi may be taken as often as you feel the need. For treating chronic kidney problems it may be taken once a day, for two to seven days, or until desired results are reached. For some, two or three times a week can be beneficial.

Contains: vitamin A, iron, minerals, and manganese.

KIDNEY

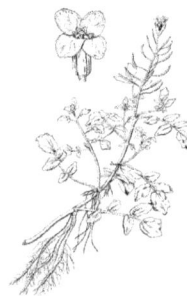

*Watercress

WATERCRESS can be a powerful herb to use for the kidneys. It treats kidney stones, liver problems, and uterine cysts. Watercress offers strength to the heart, stimulates the appetite and will increase energy. It also treats anemia, cramps, nervous problems, rheumatism, and water retention. Watercress may be taken in capsules, if it is taken as a tea, use ¼ teaspoon of Watercress herb powder to one cup of boiling water. Watercress may be taken as often as you feel the need. For treating the kidneys it may be taken once a day for two to seven days, or until desired results are reached. For some, once or twice a week can be beneficial until desired results are reached.

Contains: vitamins A, C, D, E, iron, calcium, sulphur, manganese, and copper.

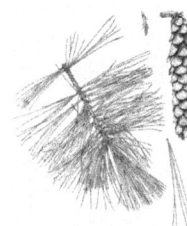

White Pine Bark

WHITE PINE BARK can be helpful for treating the kidneys. It has high medicinal qualities. It also helps with treating the lungs and whooping cough. White Pine Bark may be taken in capsules. If it is taken as a tea, use ¼ teaspoon of White Pine Bark herb powder to one cup of boiling water. White Pine Bark may be taken as often as you feel the need. For kidney problems it may be taken once or twice a day, for two to five days, or until the desired results are reached. For some, two or three times a week can be beneficial.

Contains: sodium, calcium, zinc, iodine, copper, nickel, manganese, and is very high in vitamin C.

MEMORY

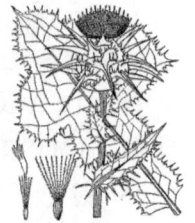

*Blessed Thistle

BLESSED THISTLE is excellent for increasing the memory. It treats senility and increases oxygen and circulation to the brain. It also treats cancer and strengthens the heart. It is helpful with treating migraine headaches. It may be taken in capsules. If it is taken as a tea, use ¼ teaspoon of Blessed Thistle herb powder to one cup of boiling water. Blessed Thistle may be taken as often as you feel the need. For chronic memory problems it may be taken two or three times a day, for two to seven days, or until desired results are reached. For some, once or twice a week will be beneficial.

Contains: B complex, calcium, iron, manganese, and potassium.

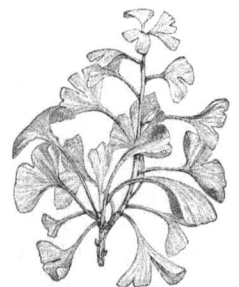

*Ginkgo

GINKGO is great for treating the memory. It treats Alzheimer's disease and dementia. It stimulates the brain and enhances mental clarity. Ginkgo treats senility and stabilizes mood swings. Ginkgo may be taken in capsules. If it is taken as a tea, use ¼ teaspoon of Ginkgo herb powder to one cup of boiling water. Ginkgo may be taken as often as you feel the need. For chronic memory problems it may be taken once or twice a day for two to ten days, or until desired results are reached. For some, once or twice a week will be beneficial.

Contains bioflavonoids.

MEMORY

Ginseng/Siberian

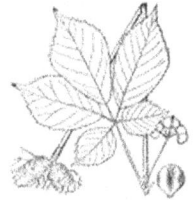

GINSENG/SIBERIAN treats loss of memory. It increases mental alertness, it treats depression, improves circulation, and slows down the aging process as well. Ginseng/Siberian also offers treatment for cancer. It may be taken in capsules. If it is taken as a tea, use ¼ teaspoon of Ginseng/Siberian herb powder to one cup of boiling water. Ginseng/Siberian may be taken as often as you feel the need. For treating the memory it may be taken once or twice a day, for two to seven days, or until desired results are reached. For some, two or three times a week until desired results are reached can be helpful.

Herbs for your blood type: Ginseng is highly beneficial for people with blood type O, A, B, and AB.

Contains: B12, sulphur, calcium, iron, sodium, and potassium.

*Goto Kola

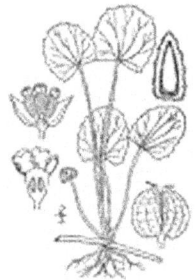

GOTO KOLA is an excellent herb for treating the loss of memory. It helps with learning problems, depression, and senility. It's great to use when there are problems with trying to concentrate. It stimulates the brain increases leg circulation, and helps to lower blood pressure. It helps to prevent nervous breakdowns. Goto Kola may be taken in capsules. If it is taken as a tea, use ¼ teaspoon of Goto Kola herb powder to one cup of boiling water. Goto Kola may be taken as often as you feel the need. For memory problems it may be taken once or twice a day, for two to ten days, or until desired results are reached. For some, two or three times a week will be beneficial.

Contains: vitamins A, G, and K, and is high in magnesium.

MEMORY

HERBS:

Rosemary

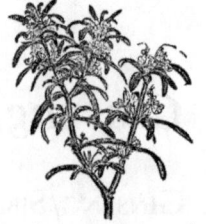

ROSEMARY can be helpful with treating the memory. It improves circulation and stimulates the brain. It is an anti-oxidant. Rosemary may elevate blood pressure for some people when taken excessively. Rosemary may be taken in capsules. If it is taken as a tea, use 1/8th teaspoon, or less of Rosemary herb powder, to one cup of boiling water. Rosemary may be taken as you feel the need. For memory problems it may be taken once or twice a day, for two to seven days, or until desired results is reached. For some once or twice a week will be helpful.

Contains: iron, sodium, potassium, zinc, phosphorus, magnesium, vitamin A and C, and is high in calcium.

NAUSEA

Basil

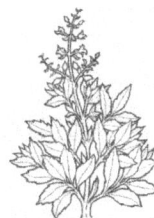

BASIL will offer relief for treating nausea. It treats uncontrollable vomiting, coughs, fevers, and nervous conditions. Basil may be kept in the kitchen and used as a spice for food preparations. It may be taken in capsules. If it is taken as a tea, use ¼ teaspoon of Basil herb powder to one cup of boiling water. Basil may be taken as often as you feel the need. For treating nausea it may be taken once or twice a day, for two to seven days, or until the desired results are reached. For some, once or twice a week can be helpful with prevention.

   Herbs for your blood type: Basil is neutral for people with blood type O, A, B, and AB.

Contains: iron, calcium, magnesium, phosphorus, vitamins A, D, and B2.

Catnip

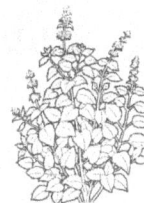

CATNIP is helpful for treating nausea. It settles the stomach, treats morning sickness, and helps to stop vomiting. Catnip also helps to treat cigarette addictions. It can also be great for treating convulsions, nervousness, and pain. It may be taken in capsules. If it is taken as a tea, use ¼ teaspoon of Catnip herb powder to one cup of boiling water. Catnip may be taken as often as you feel the need. For treating nausea it may be taken two or three times a day, for two to five days, or until desired results are reached. For some, once or twice a week can be helpful.

NAUSEA

Herbs for your blood type: Catnip is neutral for people with blood type O, B, and AB. People with blood type A should avoid this herb.

Contains: magnesium, sodium, iron, potassium, silicon, selenium, and sulphur, and is high in vitamins A, B complex, and C.

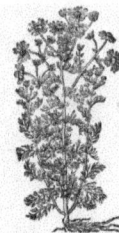

Chamomile

CHAMOMILE can be relaxing while treating nausea. It treats vomiting, menstrual cramps, and soothes stomach disorders. It also treats nervousness, and insomnia. Chamomile will increase the appetite. Chamomile may be taken in capsules, if it is taken as a tea, use ¼ teaspoon of Chamomile herb powder to one cup of boiling water. Chamomile may be taken as often as you feel the need. For treating nausea it may be taken once or twice a day, for two to five days, or until desired results are reached. For some, once or twice a week can be helpful.

Herbs for your blood type: Chamomile is highly beneficial for people with blood type A and AB. It is neutral for people with blood type O, and B.

Contains: potassium, calcium, iron, manganese, vitamin A, and zinc.

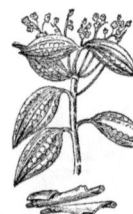

Cinnamon

CINNAMON will help to treat nausea. It calms the stomach, treats vomiting, abdominal spasms and cancer. Pregnant women should avoid Cinnamon during pregnancy. Men with prostate problems should avoid Cinnamon. Diabetics should consult a health care provider before taking Cinnamon; some herbalists say it will increase insulin activity. Cinnamon may be used as a spice in the kitchen. It may be taken in capsules. If it is taken as a tea, use ¼ teaspoon of cinnamon herb powder to one cup of boiling water. Cinnamon may be taken as often as you feel the need. For treating nausea it may be taken once or twice a day, for two to five days, or until desired results are reached. For some, once or twice a week can be helpful with prevention.

NAUSEA

Herbs for your blood type: Cinnamon is neutral for people with blood type A and blood type AB. People with blood type O and blood type B should avoid this herb.

Contains: calcium, chromium, copper, iodine, manganese, potassium, zinc, tannins, and vitamins A, B, and C.

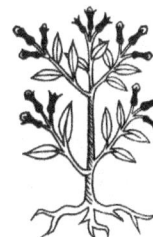

*Clove

CLOVES is highly recommended for treating nausea. It treats vomiting, bad breath, and is sometimes used to treat toothaches. It can be taken in capsules. If Cloves are taken as a tea, use ¼ teaspoon of Cloves herb powder to one cup of boiling water. Purchase Cloves from an herb store to get the greatest strength. Cloves may be taken as often as you feel the need. For treating nausea it may be taken once or twice a day, for two to five days, or until desired results are reached. For some, once or twice a week can be helpful for prevention.

Contains: sodium, potassium, calcium, magnesium, phosphorus, and vitamins A, B complex, and C.

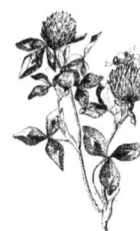

Elecampane

ELECAMPANE will assist with treating nausea. It is a stimulant that reduces water retention and increases the appetite. Elecampane will assist in reducing excessive coughing, and is helpful for treating asthma and emphysema. It is excellent for treating chronic bronchitis. It may be taken in capsules, if it is taken as a tea use ¼ teaspoon of Elecampane herb powder to one cup of boiling water. Elecampane may be taken as often as you feel the need. For treating nausea it may be taken once or twice a day, for two to three days, or until desired results are reached. For some, once or twice a week can be helpful.

Contains: sodium, calcium, and potassium.

NAUSEA

HERBS:

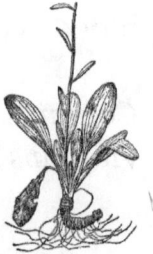

False Unicorn

FALSE UNICORN will help to treat nausea. It treats morning sickness and strengthens the reproductive and urinary organs. It also treats impotency and prostate problems, infertility, and a prolapsed uterus. False Unicorn has been known to prevent miscarriages. It will stimulate the appetite. It may be taken in capsules. If it is taken as a tea, use ¼ teaspoon of false unicorn herb powder to one cup of boiling water. False Unicorn may be taken as often as you feel the need. For treating nausea it may be taken once or twice a day for two to five days, or until desired results are reached. For some, two or three times a week will be beneficial.

Contains: vitamin C, copper, sulphur, and a small amount of zinc.

*Fennel

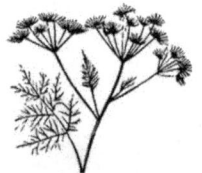

FENNEL can be excellent for treating nausea. It treats morning sickness, and can be helpful after chemotherapy and radiation treatments for cancer. It works well with other herbs and will curb the appetite. Fennel will increase urination. Fennel may elevate blood pressure for some people when taken excessively. If it must be taken use only a pinch of Fennel in combination with other herbs. Fennel may be used as a spice. Fennel may be taken in capsules. If it is taken as a tea, use ¼ teaspoon of Fennel herb powder to one cup of boiling water. Fennel may be taken as often as you feel the need. For treating nausea it may be taken once or twice a day for two to seven days, or until desired results are reached. For some, once or twice a week can help with prevention.

Contains: sodium, potassium, sulphur, and is high in vitamin A.

NAUSEA

*Ginger

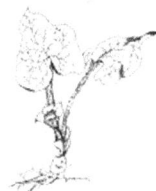

GINGER can be very beneficial for treating nausea. It is excellent for use during pregnancy. It settles the stomach and treats vomiting. Do not take aspirin while using Ginger; it will inhibit the performance of the herb. Ginger may be taken in capsules. If it is taken as a tea, use ¼ teaspoon of Ginger herb powder to one cup of boiling water. Ginger may be taken as often as you feel the need. For treating nausea/vomiting it may be taken once or twice a day, for two to five days, or until desired results are reached. For some once or twice a week can be excellent for results.

   Herbs for your blood type: Ginger is highly beneficial for people with blood type O, A, B and AB.

Contains: vitamins A, B complex, C, calcium, iron, sodium, potassium, and magnesium.

Golden Seal

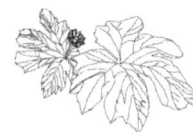

GOLDEN SEAL is helpful with treating nausea. It treats stomach problems and is strengthening to the immune system. It is helpful with menstrual disorders and has been used to stop profuse bleeding of the uterus. It can be effective at increasing blood supply to the spleen. It will reduce sugar in the blood when it is used in combination with the Licorice herb. Use Myrrh with this herb if you suffer from low blood sugar. Do not take this herb if you are pregnant. It may be taken in capsules. If it is taken as a tea, use ¼ teaspoon of Golden Seal herb powder to one cup of boiling water. Golden Seal may be taken as often as you feel the need. For nausea it may be taken once or twice a day, for two to five days, or until desired results are reached. For some, two or three times a week can be beneficial. People with high blood pressure should not use this herb more than once a week.

   Herbs for your blood type: Golden Seal is neutral for people with blood type A, B and AB. People with blood type O should avoid this herb.

Contains: calcium, potassium, iron, zinc, sodium, and vitamins A, C, B complex, and E.

NAUSEA

HERBS:

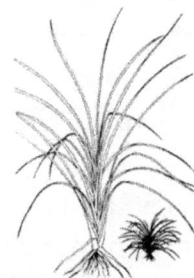

Lemon Grass

LEMON GRASS helps to treat nausea. It treats vomiting, stomach problems, and stomach cramps. Lemon grass is also great for treating fevers, kidney, and liver disorders. Lemon Grass is an excellent blood cleanser. It may be taken in capsules. If it is taken as a tea, use ¼ teaspoon of Lemon Grass herb powder to one cup of boiling water. Lemon Grass may be taken as often as you feel the need. For treating nausea it may be taken once or twice a day, for two to five days, or until desired results are reached. For some, once or twice a week can be helpful with prevention.

Contains: calcium, iron, magnesium, manganese, phosphorus, potassium, selenium, and zinc, and is high in vitamins A and C.

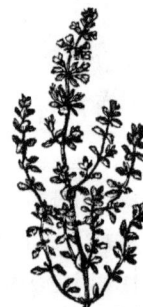

Pennyroyal

PENNYROYAL will help to relieve nausea. It treats morning sickness, migraine headaches, and toothaches. Pennyroyal is very soothing and will promote perspiration and menstruation. Do not use Pennyroyal during pregnancy it has been known to induce spontaneous abortion. It may be taken in capsules. If it is taken as a tea, use ¼ teaspoon of Pennyroyal herb powder to one cup of boiling water. Pennyroyal is best taken in combination with Kelp or Burdock. Pennyroyal may be taken as often as you feel the need. For nausea it may be taken two or three times a day until the desired results are reached.

Contains: sodium and lead.

NAUSEA

*Peppermint

PEPPERMINT is excellent for treating nausea. It settles the stomach, treats vomiting, morning sickness, motion sickness, and sea sickness. Peppermint is an energizer and will increase oxygen in the blood. It acts as a tonic to the stomach. Peppermint may be taken in capsules. If it is taken as a tea, use ¼ teaspoon of Peppermint herb powder to one cup of boiling water. Peppermint may be taken as often as you feel the need. For treating nausea it may be taken two or three times a day, for two to seven days, or until desired results are reached. For some, once or twice a week can be beneficial for prevention of nausea.

Herbs for your blood type: Peppermint is highly beneficial for people with blood type O and B. It is neutral for people with blood type A and AB.

Contains: iron, niacin, iodine, magnesium, sulphur, potassium, and vitamins A, and C.

*Red Raspberry

RED RASPBERRY is excellent to use for nausea. It can be very helpful for treating morning sickness and vomiting. Red Raspberry also enhances production of milk in the breasts of expectant mothers. Children may also use this herb for colds: for children use a smaller amount. It may be taken in capsules, if it is taken as a tea, use ¼ teaspoon of Red Raspberry herb powder to one cup of boiling water. Red Raspberry may be taken as often as you feel the need. For nausea it may be taken two or three times a day for two to five days, or until desired results are reached. For some, once or twice a week can be beneficial.

Contains: calcium, manganese, vitamins A, B, C, D, and E, Red Raspberry is very high in iron.

NAUSEA

HERBS:

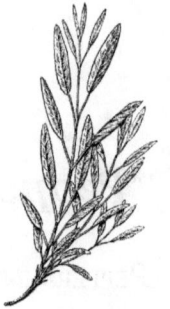

Sage

SAGE can be helpful for treating nausea. It is a good remedy for stomach troubles. It also treats mental exhaustion and improves memory. Sage will promote circulation to the heart. It will dry up saliva, and mother's breast milk. Sage may elevate blood pressure for some people when taken excessively. Sage may be used as a spice in the kitchen. It may be taken in capsules. If it is taken as a tea, use ¼ teaspoon of Sage herb powder to one cup of boiling water. Sage may be taken as often as you feel the need. For nausea it may be taken once or twice a day, for two to five days, or until desired results are reached. For some, once or twice a week can be helpful.

Herbs for your blood type: Sage is highly beneficial for people with blood type B. It is neutral for people with blood type O, A, and AB.

Contains: sodium, sulphur, vitamins A, B complex, and C.

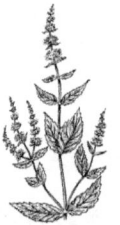

*Spearmint

SPEARMINT is excellent for treating nausea. It treats vomiting, morning sickness, and nervousness. It is an excellent herb to use for the sickest person and gentle enough for babies with colic. Spearmint can be taken in capsules. If it is taken as a tea, use ¼ teaspoon of Spearmint herb powder to one cup of boiling water. Spearmint may be taken as often as you feel the need. For nausea it may be taken two or three times a day for two to five days, or until desired results are reached. For some, two or three times a week can be beneficial.

Herbs for your blood type: Spearmint is neutral for people with blood type O, A, B and AB.

Contains: calcium, iron, sulphur, iodine, potassium, magnesium, vitamin A, C, and B complex.

NAUSEA

White Oak Bark

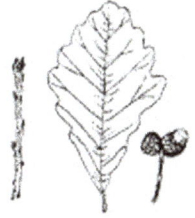

WHITE OAK BARK will help to settle the stomach from nausea. It will help to stop vomiting. It is also excellent for stopping bleeding of the teeth. White Oak Bark will increase urine flow, and it gives support to the bladder. It treats PMS and it can be useful for treating external and internal bleeding. White Oak Bark should be taken in combination with Burdock or Kelp. White Oak Bark may elevate blood pressure for some people when taken excessively. White Oak Bark may be taken in capsules. If it is taken as a tea, use ¼ teaspoon of White Oak Bark herb powder to one cup of boiling water. White Oak Bark may be taken as often as you feel the need. For nausea it may be taken once or twice a day, for two to five days, or until desired results are reached. For some, once or twice a week can be helpful for prevention.

Contains: sodium, cobalt, lead, iodine, potassium, calcium, sulphur, and vitamin B12.

Wild Yam

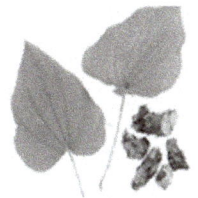

WILD YAM will help to relieve nausea. It treats irritation and inflammation in the stomach, it treats morning sickness. It also treats Addison's disease, increases energy, assists with weight loss, and gastrointestinal problems. It soothes the nerves, and treats liver and urinary problems. Wild Yam will promote perspiration. Wild Yam may be taken in capsules. If it is taken as a tea, use ¼ teaspoon of Wild Yam herb powder to one cup of boiling water. Wild Yam may be taken as often as you feel the need. For nausea it may be taken once or twice a day, for two to seven days, or until desired results are reached. For some, once a week can be beneficial.

Contains: vitamins A, B complex, C, iron, potassium, sodium, phosphorus, calcium, silicon, magnesium, and manganese.

PNEUMONIA

HERBS:

Anise

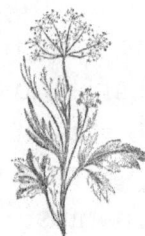

ANISE can assist with treating pneumonia. It treats hard dry coughs, asthma, and emphysema. Anise will stimulate the appetite, it is an excellent herb for treating indigestion and colds. Anise has high estrogens levels. It is a stimulant for the heart, liver, brains, and lungs. Anise can also be used as a spice in the kitchen. It may be taken in capsules. If Anise is taken as a tea, use ¼ teaspoon of Anise herb powder to one cup of boiling water. Anise may be taken as often as you feel the need. For treating pneumonia it may be taken two or three times a day, for three to ten days, or until desired results are reached. For some, two or three times a week can be helpful.

Contains: iron, calcium, potassium, and magnesium, and B vitamins.

*Bee Propolis

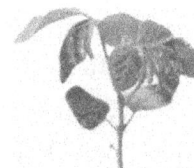

BEE PROPOLIS can be excellent for treating pneumonia. It is a powerful anti-viral herb. It stimulates the immune system and treats a variety of viral infections that are similar to pneumonia. It treats intestinal and stomach ulcers, and increases new cell growth. It has been used to reduce high blood pressure. Bee Propolis may be taken in capsules. If it is taken as a tea, use ¼ teaspoon of Bee Propolis herb powder to one cup of boiling water. Bee Propolis may be taken as often as you feel the need. For pneumonia it may be taken once or twice a day for three to ten days

PNEUMONIA

at a time, or until the desired results are reached. For some, once or twice a week can be beneficial.

Contains: iron, zinc, copper magnesium, silicon, and manganese.

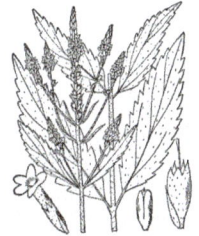

Blue Vervain

BLUE VERVAIN can be helpful for treating pneumonia. It helps to clear upper respiratory and inflammation of the lungs, it treats lung congestion, consumption, and whooping cough. Blue Vervain offers a calm and tranquilizing effect on the body. Using large amounts of this herb at once may cause vomiting. It may be taken in capsules. If it is taken as a tea, use ¼ teaspoon of Blue Vervain herb powder to one cup of boiling water. Blue Vervain may be taken as often as you feel the need. For treating pneumonia it may be taken once or twice a day for three to five days at a time, or until desired results are reached. For some, once or twice a week can be helpful.

Contains: vitamin C, calcium, manganese, and vitamin E.

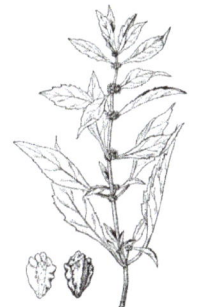

Bugleweed

BUGLEWEED will assist with treating pneumonia. It offers success with reducing hemorrhaging, and fluids in the lungs. It also treats pain, calms the nerves, and soothes the heart. Bugleweed lowers the pulse and stabilizes an irregular heartbeat. It may be taken in capsules. If it is taken as a tea, use ¼ teaspoon of Bugleweed herb powder to one cup of boiling water. Bugleweed may be taken as often as you feel the need. For pneumonia it may be taken once or twice a day for three to seven days, or until desired results are reached. For some, once or twice a week can be helpful.

Content: vitamin information unknown.

PNEUMONIA

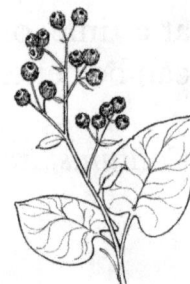

Burdock

BURDOCK will help to treat pneumonia. It treats inflammation in the lungs, coughs, tuberculosis, cancer, bursitis, and constipation. It also reduces fluid retention and swelling in the body. **An excessive amount of Burdock taken at once, may cause vomiting**. It may be taken in capsules. If it is taken as a tea, use ¼ teaspoon of Burdock herb powder to one cup of boiling water. Burdock may be taken as often as you feel the need. For pneumonia it may be taken once or twice a day for three to seven days at a time, or until desired results are reached. For some once or twice a week will be beneficial.

Herbs for your blood type: Burdock is highly beneficial for people with blood type A and AB. It is neutral for people with blood type B. People with blood type O should avoid this herb it will cause excessive blood thinning and excessive bleeding for them.

Contains: vitamins A, B complex, C, and E, iron, zinc, iodine, copper, and sulphur.

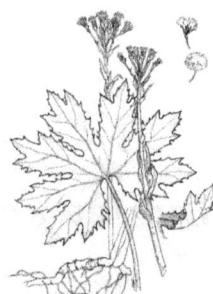

Coltsfoot

COLTSFOOT can be helpful with treating pneumonia. It treats inflammation in the lungs, asthma, bronchitis, dry coughs, and mucus. **Coltsfoot may elevate blood pressure for some people when taken excessively.** Coltsfoot may be taken in capsules, if it is taken as a tea, use ¼ teaspoon of Coltsfoot herb powder to one cup of boiling water. Coltsfoot may be taken as often as you feel the need. For pneumonia it may be taken once or twice a day, for three to seven days, or until desired results are achieved. For some, once or twice a week can be beneficial.

Herbs for your blood type: Coltsfoot is highly beneficial for people with blood type A. People with blood type O, B and AB. should avoid this herb.

PNEUMONIA

HERBS:

Contains: a high amount of vitamins A and C; calcium, potassium, manganese, copper, zinc; vitamins P, B12, and B6.

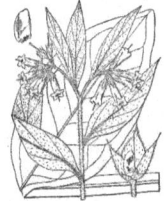

Comfrey

COMFREY can assist with treating pneumonia. It removes mucus from the lungs, treats emphysema, and tuberculosis. Comfrey stimulates new cell growth and promotes healing throughout the body. It may be taken in capsules, if it is taken as a tea, use ¼ teaspoon of Comfrey herb powder to one cup of boiling water. Comfrey may be taken as often as you feel the need. For pneumonia it may be taken once or twice a day, for three to ten days, or until desired results are reached. For some, two or three days a week can be helpful.

Contains: vitamins A, C, iron, sulphur, copper, zinc, and magnesium. Comfrey is very high in calcium, potassium, and protein.

*Elder Flower

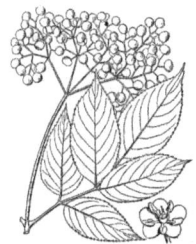

ELDER FLOWER can be excellent for treating pneumonia. It clears the lungs, reduces fever, treats asthma, bronchitis, and acts a sedative while reducing pain. It may be taken in capsules. If it is taken as a tea, use ¼ teaspoon of Elder Flower herb powder to one cup of boiling water. Elder Flower may be taken as often as you feel the need. For pneumonia it may be taken once or twice a day, for three to ten days, or until desired results are reached.

Herbs for your blood type: Elder Flower is neutral for people of blood type O, A, B and AB.

Contains: vitamins A and C.

PNEUMONIA

Eucalyptus

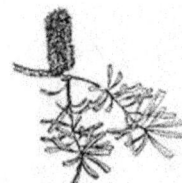

EUCALYPTUS treats pneumonia; respiratory infections, and congestion in the lungs. Eucalyptus oil can be used as a steam inhalant, or it may be rubbed on the chest and back for relief to the lungs. Use it as a vapor

Ginger

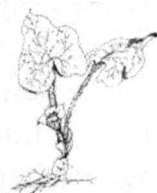

GINGER will help to treat pneumonia. It treats chronic bronchitis and influenza. It settles the stomach and it is great for treating whooping cough. **Do not take aspirin while using Ginger; it will inhibit the performance of the herb.** Ginger is best found in the produce section of the grocery market and may be used in foods as a spice. Ginger may be taken in capsules. Or, use ¼ teaspoon of Ginger herb powder to one cup of boiling water. Ginger may be taken as often as you feel the need. For pneumonia it may be taken two or three times a day for three to seven days, or until the desired results are reached. For some, once or twice a day will offer relief.

Herbs for your blood type: Ginger is highly beneficial for people with blood type O, A, B and AB. Contains: vitamins A, B complex, C, calcium, iron, sodium, potassium, and magnesium.

Irish Moss

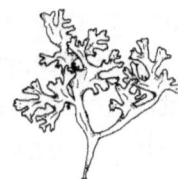

IRISH MOSS can be effective with treating pneumonia. It treats respiratory problems, chronic lung problems, and bronchitis. Irish Moss clears the lungs and rids the body of extra fluids; it would be wise to use a very small amount of this herb and increase it as you feel the need. If Irish Moss is taken as a tea, use a small pinch in

PNEUMONIA

combination with other herbs. Use ¼ teaspoon to one cup of boiling water. Irish Moss may be taken as often as you feel the need. For pneumonia it may be taken once or twice a day, for two to five days, or until the desired results are reached. For some, two or three times a week will offer relief.

Contains: vitamins A, D, E, F, and K, sodium, calcium potassium, sulphur, and is very high in iodine.

*Lobelia

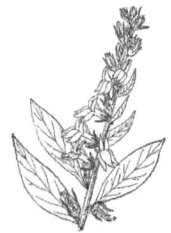

LOBELIA will be very effective in treating pneumonia. It treats chronic lung problems, fevers, pleurisy, and bronchitis. Lobelia relaxes the entire system and increases urine flow. It may be taken in capsules. If it is taken as a tea, use ¼ teaspoon of Lobelia herb powder to one cup of boiling water. Lobelia may be taken as often as you feel the need. For pneumonia it may be taken once or twice a day, for three to seven days, or until desired results are reached. For some, two or three times a week can offer desired results.

Contains: iron, copper, sodium, sulphur, cobalt, lead, and selenium.

LOTS OF WATER SHOULD BE TAKEN WITH LOBELIA.

*Marshmallow

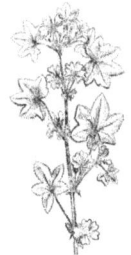

MARSHMALLOW is an excellent herb for treating pneumonia. It soothes the mucous membranes, treats asthma, and emphysema. **Marshmallow may elevate blood pressure for some people when taken excessively.** Marshmallow may be taken in capsules. If it is taken as a tea, use ¼ teaspoon of Marshmallow herb powder to one cup of boiling water. Marshmallow may be taken as often as you feel the need. For pneumonia it may be taken once or twice a day, for three to ten days, or until

PNEUMONIA

HERBS:

desired results are reached. For some, two or three times a week will be beneficial for desired results.

Do not confuse Marshmallow herb with the candy like marshmallow found in the food section of the market.

Contains: sodium, iodine, B complex, pantothenic acid, and is high in calcium, zinc, and iron.

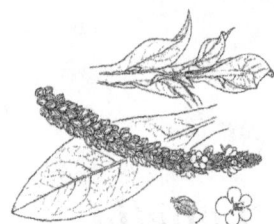

Mullein

MULLEIN will be helpful for treating pneumonia. It clears the lungs when they are swollen or bleeding. It treats congestion and respiratory problems. **Mullein is best taken at bedtime because it will cause sleepiness. It may be taken in capsules.** If it is taken as a tea, use ¼ teaspoon of Mullein herb powder to one cup of boiling water. Mullein may be taken as often as you feel the need. For pneumonia it may be taken once or twice a day, for three to ten days, or until desired results are reached. For some, once or twice a week can be beneficial.

Herbs for your blood type: Mullein is neutral for people with blood type O and A. People with blood type B and AB should avoid this herb.

Contains: magnesium, potassium, and sulphur. Mullein is very high in iron.

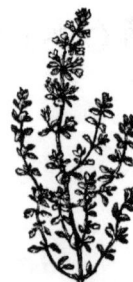

Pennyroyal

PENNYROYAL will assist with treating pneumonia. It treats lung infections, bronchitis, excessive mucus, convulsion, and flu. Pennyroyal is very soothing and will promote perspiration and menstruation. **Do not use Pennyroyal during pregnancy, it has been known to induce spontaneous abortion.** It may be taken in capsules. If it is taken as a tea, use ¼ teaspoon of Pennyroyal herb powder to one cup of boiling water. Pennyroyal should be taken in combination with Kelp or Burdock. Pennyroyal may be taken as often as you feel the need. For pneumonia it may be taken once or twice a day, for three to seven days, or until desired results are reached. For some, two or three times a week will be beneficial.

PNEUMONIA

HERBS:

Contains: sodium and lead.

*Pleurisy Root

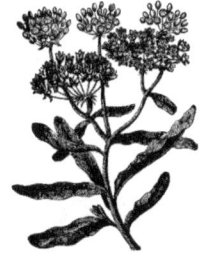

PLEURISY ROOT is an excellent herb for treating pneumonia; it treats lung congestion, fevers, and mucus. It clears the lungs and improves oxygen intake. It helps to clear thick mucus, inflammation, and phlegm. Vitamin C should be taken when using this herb. Pleurisy Root relaxes the whole body. **Pleurisy Root is not recommended for children. It may cause vomiting when taken excessively. Do not use Pleurisy during pregnancy it may induce spontaneous abortion. Do not use while breast-feeding. Large amounts of Pleurisy Root may be very toxic. Do not use Pleurisy if there is a history of heart disease, or certain types of cancer.** It may be taken in capsules, if it is taken as a tea, use ¼ teaspoon of Pleurisy Root herb powder to one cup of boiling water. Pleurisy Root may be taken as often as you feel the need. For pneumonia it may be taken once a day for two to ten days, or until desired results are reached. For some, once or twice a week can be beneficial.

Sage

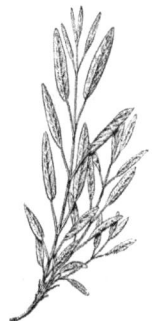

SAGE can be helpful for treating pneumonia. It treats lung problems, fevers, and flu. It can help with treating night sweats as well. It also helps to improve memory and treat some forms of mental illness. Sage will dry up saliva, perspiration, and mother's milk. **Sage may elevate blood pressure for some people when taken excessively.** It may be taken in capsules. If it is taken as a tea, use ¼ teaspoon of Sage herb powder to one cup of boiling water. Sage may be taken as often as you feel the need. For pneumonia it may be taken once or twice a day, for three to seven days, or until desired results are reached. For some, two or three time a week can be helpful.

Herbs for your blood type: Sage is highly beneficial for people with blood type B. It is neutral for people with blood type O, A, and AB.

PNEUMONIA

HERBS:

Contains: sodium, sulphur, vitamins A, B complex, and C.

*Seneca

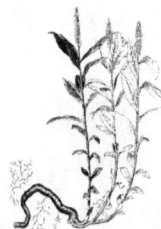

SENECA is great for treating pneumonia. It treats lung congestion, acute bronchitis, and chronic catarrh. It treats convulsion and inflammation of the mucus membrane. Seneca may be taken in capsules, if it is taken as a tea add ¼ teaspoon of Seneca powder herb to one cup of boiling water. Seneca may be taken as often as you feel the need. For pneumonia it may be taken once or twice a day for two to seven days, or until desires results are reached. For some, once or twice a week can be helpful.

Contains: iron, lead, tin, aluminum, and magnesium.

Yarrow

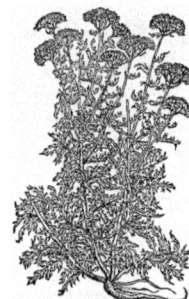

YARROW can be helpful for treating pneumonia. It treats hemorrhaging lungs, mucous membrane, and chronic catarrh. Yarrow may be found in the produce section of the market. Yarrow may be taken in capsules. If it is taken as a tea, use ¼ teaspoon of Yarrow herb powder to one cup of boiling water. Yarrow may be taken as often as you feel the need. For pneumonia it may be taken once or twice a day, for two to ten days, or until desired results are reached. For some, two or three times a week can be helpful.

Contains: iron, iodine, manganese, copper, potassium, and vitamins A, C, E, F, and K.

SCIATICA

*Burdock

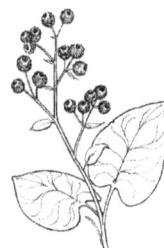

BURDOCK is excellent for treating sciatica pain. It also treats arthritis, bursitis, and gout. Burdock is excellent for treating rheumatism, itching, and swelling. It also treats fluid retention, hemorrhoids, herpes, and cleans the lymphatic system. It increases urine flow. Burdock is useful in treating a variety of illnesses and sciatica pain is one at the top of the list. It may be taken in capsules, if it is taken as a tea use ¼ teaspoon of Burdock herb powder to one cup of boiling water. Burdock may be taken as often as you feel the need. For sciatica pain it may be taken once or twice a day, for three to seven days, or until desired results are reached. For some, once or twice a week will be beneficial. An excessive amount of Burdock at once may cause vomiting.

Herbs for your blood type: Burdock is highly beneficial for people with blood type A and AB. It is neutral for people with blood type B. People with blood type O should avoid this herb it will cause excessive blood thinning and excessive bleeding.

Contains: vitamins A, B complex, C, and E, iron, zinc, and sulphur.

Horseradish

HORSERADISH will be helpful in treating the sciatic nerve. It also treats arthritis, neuralgia, poor circulation, digestive disorders, the liver, and the spleen. Horseradish stimulates the appetite. It may be taken in capsules. If it is taken as a tea, use ¼ teaspoon of Horseradish herb powder to one cup of boiling water. Horseradish may

SCIATICA

be taken as often as you feel the need. For sciatic nerve pain it may be taken once or twice a day, for three to seven days, or until desired results are reached. For some, once or twice a week can be helpful.

Contains: vitamins A, B complex, iron, calcium, sodium, and phosphorus.

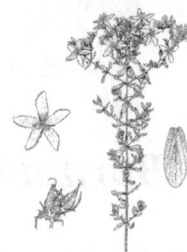

St. John's Wort

ST. JOHN'S WORT can be useful as treatment for sciatic pain. Use it as a liniment; it relieves pain when applied externally as a poultice to the sciatica, or spine area St. John's Wort removes malignant and benign growths. Fair skin people should stay out of the sunlight while taking this herb. It may be taken in capsules. If it is taken as a tea, use ¼ teaspoon of St. Johns Wort to one cup of boiling water. St. John's Wort may be taken as often as you feel the need. For sciatic pain it may be taken once or twice a day, for two to seven days, or until desired results are reached. For some, once or twice a week can offer desired results.

Herbs for your blood type: St. John's Wort is highly beneficial for people with blood type A. It is neutral for people with blood type B and AB. People with blood type O should avoid this herb.

Contains bioflavonoids.

SCIATICA

*Thyme

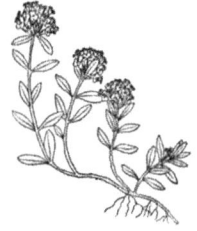

THYME is excellent to us for treating the sciatic nerve. It also treats shingles, spasms, sprains, and shortness of breath. It has been known to kill worms in the stomach. Thyme may elevate blood pressure for some when taken excessively. Thyme can be kept in the kitchen and used as a spice. It may be taken in capsules. If it is taken as a tea, use ¼ teaspoon of Thyme herb powder to one cup of boiling water. Thyme may be taken as often as you feel the need. For sciatica pain it may be taken once or twice a day, for two to five days, or until desired results are reached. For some, once or twice a week can be beneficial.

Herbs for your blood type: Thyme is highly beneficial for people with blood type O and B. It is neutral for people with blood type A and AB.

Contains: sodium, iodine sulphur, and vitamins C, and D.

Wintergreen

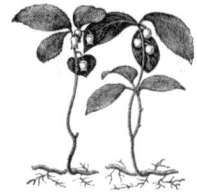

WINTERGREEN will help to relieve pain to the sciatic nerve. It also treats over exhausted muscles and joints. It is most effective when taken internally and applied externally at the same time, to treat aches and lower back pain. It treats gout, inflammation, rheumatism and urinary problems. It may be taken in capsules. It is taken as a tea, use ¼ teaspoon of Wintergreen herb powder to one cup of boiling water. Wintergreen may be taken as often as you feel the need. For treating sciatic pain it may be taken once or twice a day, for two to five days, or until desired results are reached. For some, once or twice a week can be helpful.

Vitamin Content unknown.

BIBLIOGRAPHY

Annette and Richard Bloch
FIGHTING CANCER
R. A. Bloch Cancer Foundation – Publisher
4410 Main Street, Kansas City, Missouri 64111

Dr. Peter J. D'Adamo – Catherine Whitney
EAT RIGHT FOR YOUR TYPE
G. P. Putnam's Sons
Publishers 200 Madison Avenue
New York, NY 10016

Jack Ritchason, N.D.
THE LITTLE HERB ENCYCLOPEDIA
Third Edition

James F. Balch, M.D. – Phyllis A. Balch, C.N.C.
NUTRITIONAL HEALING
Avery Publishing Group

Jeanne Rose's Herbal
HERB'S & THINGS
Perigee Books
The Berkley Publishing Group

John B. Lust, N.D. D.B.M.
THE HERB BOOK
Bantam Books
New York – Toronto – London, Sydney- Auckland

Louise Tenney, M. H.
TODAY'S HERBAL HEALTH
Forth Edition
Woodland Publishing Inc.

Michael Castleman
THE HEALING HERBS
Bantam Books
New York – Toronto – London – Sydney - Auckland

* 9 7 8 0 6 1 5 1 9 8 1 2 5 *